Fix Your Stress Biology

Also by Ya-Ling J. Liou D.C.

Put Out the Fire: "It Never Used to Hurt When I...?!"
(The Everyday Pain Guide, Volume 1)

Fix the Fire Damage: Your go-to guide when pain first strikes
(The Everyday Pain Guide, Volume 2)

Fix Your Body Mechanics: Companion Manual & Journal
(The Everyday Pain Guide Workbooks #1)

Fix Your Body Chemistry: Companion Manual & Journal
(The Everyday Pain Guide Workbooks #2)

Fix Your Stress Biology: Companion Manual & Journal
(The Everyday Pain Guide Workbooks #3)

The Everyday Pain Guide WORKBOOKS

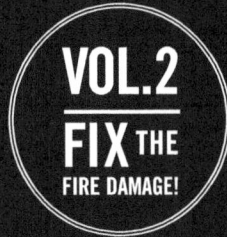

VOL.2

FIX THE
FIRE DAMAGE!

Fix Your Stress Biology

COMPANION MANUAL & JOURNAL

YA-LING J. LIOU, D.C.

Artwork by SANDY JOHNSON

RETURN TO HEALTH PRESS

SEATTLE, WA

FIX YOUR STRESS BIOLOGY COMPANION MANUAL & JOURNAL
(THE EVERYDAY PAIN GUIDE WORKBOOKS #3)
© 2025 Ya-Ling J. Liou, D.C.
All rights reserved.

Published by Return to Health Press, Seattle, WA
Ya-Ling J. Liou, D.C., is a chiropractic physician in Seattle, WA
www.returntohealthpress.com

Notice
The information, techniques and suggestions contained in this book are not intended as a substitute for individual medical care. All matters regarding your health require medical supervision. Consult your health care professional before performing any exercise or taking any dietary supplement referenced in this book. Neither the author, nor the publisher, contributors or editors shall be liable or responsible for any loss, damage or risk arising, directly or indirectly, from the use and application of any of the contents of this book.

Cover Design by VMC Art & Design, LLC
Interior Design by VMC Art & Design, LLC
Image & Diagram Credits: 1983 Wong-Baker FACES Foundation. www.wongbakerfaces.org
Illustrations by Sandy Johnson

First Edition, 2025
Printed in the United States of America

ISBN: 978-0-9913094-6-7

CONTENTS

Author's Note

For best results, make sure to seek care as soon as possible and/or in conjunction with these strategies. Always check with a healthcare provider first.

SURPRISE PAIN?

Neck/Shoulder

Mid Back/Torso/Ribs

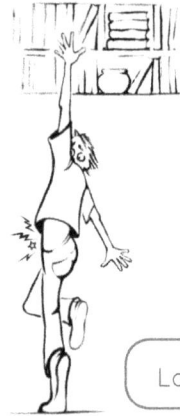

Neck

Low Back

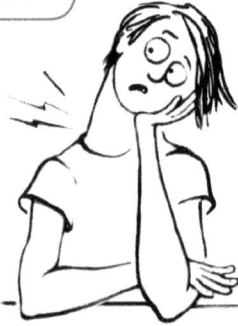

Shoulder/Upper Back

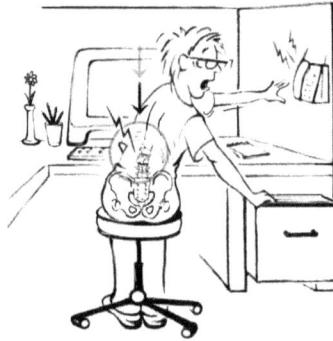

Hip/Buttock/Thigh

Low Back/Hip

☑ BODY MECHANICS ACTION PLANS

☑ BODY CHEMISTRY ACTION PLAN

➡ **STRESS BIOLOGY ACTION PLAN**

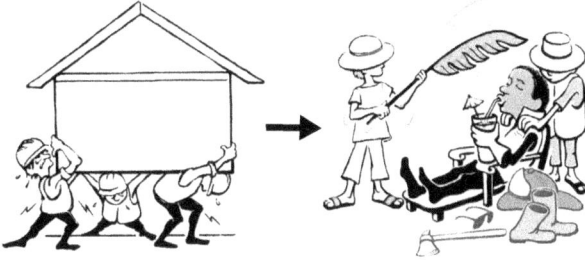

1. RELEASE

- *Mechanical Strain*
- *Body Chemistry Garbage*
- **Emotional Stress Triggers**

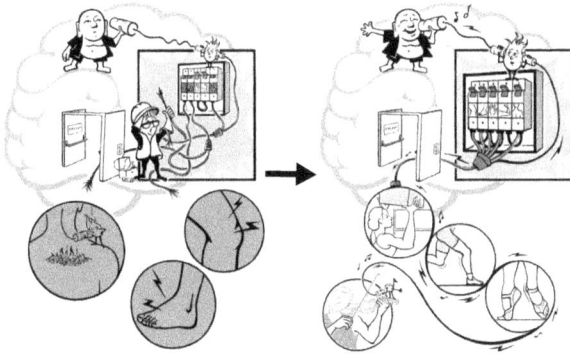

2. RETRAIN

- *Body-Brain Connection*
- *Garbage Journeys*
- **Nervous System**

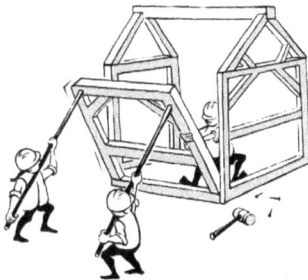

3. REINFORCE

- *Mechanical Structure*
- *Garbage Elimination*
- **Low-Stress Biology**

IS IT TIME TO EXPLORE THE STRESS BIOLOGY ACTION PLAN?

➤ Did your everyday pain episode start around the same time as a big life change?

    ☐ Yes

    ☐ No

➤ Did you already explore the Body Mechanics and/or Body Chemistry Action Plans and feel relief, but your pain keeps returning?

    ☐ Yes

    ☐ No

➤ Do you also have any of the following:

    ☐ Unusual irritability or impatience

    ☐ Feelings of overwhelm

    ☐ Missing sense of humor

    ☐ Lack of motivation

    ☐ Other _____

If you answered "yes" to any or all of the above, it's a good time to explore this next section about stress biology.

Notes:

"It's not stress that kills us, it's our reaction to it."

—Hans Selye

My Release & Retrain Action Steps

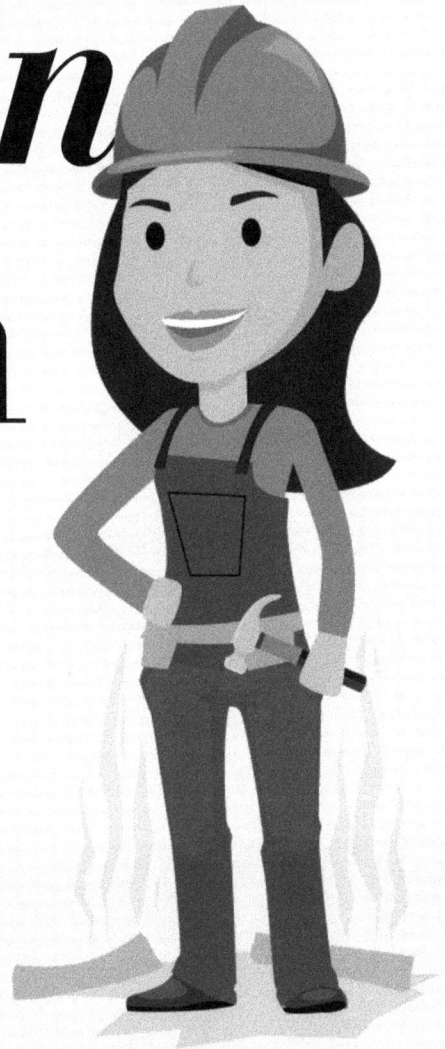

THE CHECK IN

How are you feeling?

TODAY'S DATE: _____

PAIN LOCATION:
(circle one)

Neck   Neck/Shoulder   Shoulder/Upper Back   Mid Back/Torso/Ribs

Low Back   Low Back/Hip   Hip/Buttock/Thigh

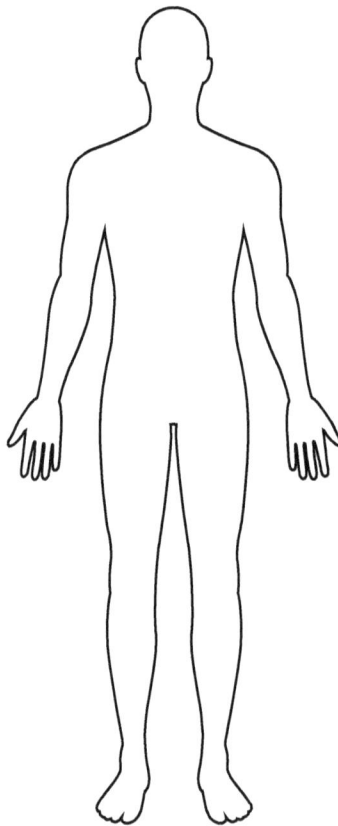

Use this figure to color or shade-in the area of your pain however you like.

HOW MUCH PAIN TODAY?

Circle the face below that best expresses your discomfort:

Wong-Baker FACES® Pain Rating Scale

0	2	4	6	8	10
No Pain	A Little Pain	A Little More Pain	Even More Pain	A Whole Lot Of Pain	Worst Pain

Notes:

_____

_____

_____

_____

_____

_____

_____

_____

_____

What coping pitfalls do I want to deal with?
(circle all that apply)

Toxic Positivity   Toxic Distraction   Overanalysis

Unchecked Venting

Other/More Details: _____

_____

_____

_____

_____

_____

My stress-triggering food:
(circle all that apply)

Saturated Fats   Sugars   Sweet Treats   Salty Snacks

Fried Food   Caffeine   Processed Foods

Other/More Details: _____

_____

_____

_____

_____

_____

My sleep is affected by:
(circle all that apply)

Waking Up   Bedtime   Sleep Quality

Other/More Details: _____

_____

_____

_____

_____

_____

How does play and exercise factor into my stress response?

_____

_____

_____

_____

_____

_____

_____

My Five Senses:

(Write down a few things that have both positive and negative reactions.)

Sight   Positive: _____

_____

_____

Negative: _____

_____

_____

Smell   Positive: _____

_____

_____

Negative: _____

_____

_____

Sound Positive: _____

_____

_____

Negative: _____

_____

_____

Touch Positive: _____

_____

_____

Negative: _____

_____

_____

Taste Positive: _____

_____

Negative: _____

_____

My Posture In Response To Stress:

(Use this space to draw or write down what your posture looks like.)

What relationships affect my stress?
(circle all that apply)

Home   Work   Family   Friends

Other: _____

More Details: _____

_____

_____

_____

_____

What pain biases do I want to deal with?
(circle all that apply)

Body Weight   Hunching Posture   Arthritis

Disc Disease   Sciatica

Other/More Details: _____

_____

_____

_____

_____

_____

RELEASE & RETRAIN!

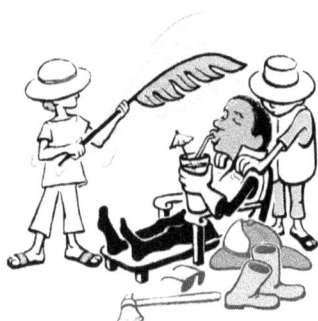 &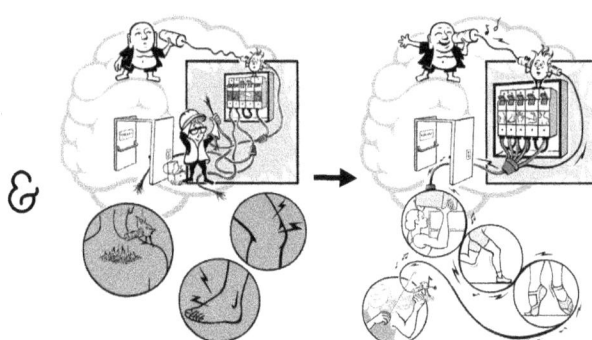

RELEASE   RETRAIN

Q: *What* are you releasing and retraining?

A: **Your emotional stress triggers and your nervous system**

Q: *How* are you releasing your emotional stress triggers and retraining
your nervous system?

A: **Choose healthy coping, use your five senses, tend to your sleep,
play and relationships, strengthen safety postures and reconsider
your biases**

➤ Go to the book for more: *Fix the Fire Damage*, pages 484 – 511

➤ Listen to the podcast: *Conversations About Everyday Pai*n, Season 2,
Episodes 52 - 57

NEXT STEPS:

1. Release toxic coping with healthy alternatives

2. Retrain your nervous system using your five senses

3. Retrain your glucose metabolism through food, sleep, play, and relationships

4. Release fear postures by strengthening safety postures

5. Retrain your health and wellness biases

RELEASE TOXIC POSITIVITY

What emotions come up when you're in pain?

(Circle one or write in your emotion.)

Fear   Anger   Guilt

Other: _____

Tell me more:

_____

_____

_____

_____

_____

_____

_____

_____

_____

_____

_____

_____

_____

_____

_____

_____

_____

_____

_____

_____

_____

_____

RELEASE TOXIC POSITIVITY

Your body is not trying to trick you. Your pain is an important message.

What is the message?

_____

_____

_____

_____

_____

_____

_____

How can you show your body that you're listening, and you care?

_____

_____

_____

_____

_____

_____

_____

Remember, your pain is not permanent. But right now, it's okay to feel angry, frustrated or scared.

Let it all out here and tell me more:

_____

_____

_____

_____

_____

_____

_____

_____

_____

_____

_____

_____

_____

My Coping Journal

Toxic Positivity

_____

_____

_____

_____

_____

_____

_____

_____

_____

_____

_____

_____

_____

_____

_____

_____

_____

_____

_____

_____

_____

_____

_____

_____

_____

_____

_____

_____

_____

_____

_____

_____

MY COPING JOURNAL: TOXIC POSITIVITY

RELEASE TOXIC DISTRACTION

What or who can you say "no" to...

TODAY

➤ _____

➤ _____

➤ _____

➤ _____

➤ _____

THIS WEEK

➤ _____

➤ _____

➤ _____

➤ _____

➤ _____

RELEASE TOXIC DISTRACTION

THIS MONTH

➤ _____

➤ _____

➤ _____

➤ _____

➤ _____

THIS YEAR

➤ _____

➤ _____

➤ _____

➤ _____

➤ _____

RELEASE TOXIC DISTRACTION

Now that you have said "no" to something or someone, what will you do with that time and energy instead?

_____

_____

_____

_____

_____

_____

_____

_____

_____

_____

_____

_____

_____

_____

_____

_____

_____

_____

_____

_____

_____

_____

_____

SUGGESTIONS:

➤ Try a meditation app

➤ Set your alarm for 10-15 min. of just sitting silently looking out the window or resting your eyelids closed. Notice your breath. Notice your body temperature. Let your belly relax.

➤ Put "me-time" on your calendar once a week or once a month. Get a massage, take a walk, daydream, nap in the middle of the day, get a facial, talk to a friend, explore crafting or hobby time.

5-10 Minute Daily Check-In

DAY 1

TODAY'S DATE: _____

Now that you are refocusing your energy and time, scan your body for physical sensations and emotional states. Describe those here:

_____

_____

_____

_____

_____

_____

_____

_____

_____

_____

_____

_____

_____

_____

DAY 2

TODAY'S DATE: _____

Now that you are refocusing your energy and time, scan your body for physical sensations and emotional states. Describe those here:

_____

_____

_____

_____

_____

_____

_____

_____

_____

_____

_____

_____

_____

DAY 3

TODAY'S DATE: _____

Now that you are refocusing your energy and time, scan your body
for physical sensations and emotional states. Describe those here:

_____

_____

_____

_____

_____

_____

_____

_____

_____

_____

_____

_____

DAY 4

TODAY'S DATE: _____

Now that you are refocusing your energy and time, scan your body for physical sensations and emotional states. Describe those here:

_____

_____

_____

_____

_____

_____

_____

_____

_____

_____

_____

_____

_____

DAY 5

TODAY'S DATE: _____

Now that you are refocusing your energy and time, scan your body for physical sensations and emotional states. Describe those here:

_____

_____

_____

_____

_____

_____

_____

_____

_____

_____

_____

DAY 6

TODAY'S DATE: _____

Now that you are refocusing your energy and time, scan your body for physical sensations and emotional states. Describe those here:

_____

_____

_____

_____

_____

_____

_____

_____

_____

_____

_____

_____

_____

DAY 7

TODAY'S DATE: _____

Now that you are refocusing your energy and time, scan your body for physical sensations and emotional states. Describe those here:

_____

_____

_____

_____

_____

_____

_____

_____

_____

_____

_____

_____

_____

Schedule A Digital Detox

RELEASE TOXIC DISTRACTION: DIGITAL DETOX

Replace doomscrolling with moving your body.

Whether for one day, a week, or a full week every few months, taking a break from mindlessly doomscrolling through your phone or staring at a screen can help to reset your mood chemicals., A break from social media, TV/videos, streaming, or gaming can help your brain remember how to access your feel-good chemicals more organically. (Refer pages 488-489 in *Fix the Fire Damage* for more information.)

Jot down a few ideas about what you can do during your digital detox.

➤ _____

➤ _____

➤ _____

➤ _____

➤ _____

SUGGESTIONS:

➤ A short dance break
➤ Yoga
➤ A gentle walk
➤ A bike ride

Replace doomscrolling with moving your body.

TODAY'S DATE: _____

What activity did you choose?

_____

_____

_____

How did it feel?

_____

_____

_____

_____

_____

_____

_____

_____

RELEASE TOXIC DISTRACTION: DIGITAL DETOX

Replace doomscrolling with moving your body.

TODAY'S DATE: _____

What activity did you choose?

_____

_____

_____

How did it feel?

_____

_____

_____

_____

_____

_____

_____

_____

Replace doomscrolling with moving your body.

TODAY'S DATE: _____

What activity did you choose?

_____

_____

_____

How did it feel?

_____

_____

_____

_____

_____

_____

_____

_____

RELEASE TOXIC DISTRACTION: DIGITAL DETOX

Replace doomscrolling with moving your body.

TODAY'S DATE: _____

What activity did you choose?

_____

_____

_____

How did it feel?

_____

_____

_____

_____

_____

_____

_____

_____

Replace doomscrolling with moving your body.

TODAY'S DATE: _____

What activity did you choose?

_____

_____

_____

How did it feel?

_____

_____

_____

_____

_____

_____

_____

_____

RELEASE TOXIC DISTRACTION: DIGITAL DETOX

Replace doomscrolling with moving your body.

TODAY'S DATE: _____

What activity did you choose?

_____

_____

_____

How did it feel?

_____

_____

_____

_____

_____

_____

_____

_____

Replace doomscrolling with moving your body.

TODAY'S DATE: _____

What activity did you choose?

_____

_____

_____

How did it feel?

_____

_____

_____

_____

_____

_____

_____

_____

RELEASE TOXIC DISTRACTION: DIGITAL DETOX

Replace doomscrolling with moving your body.

TODAY'S DATE: _____

What activity did you choose?

_____

_____

_____

How did it feel?

_____

_____

_____

_____

_____

_____

_____

_____

RELEASE OVERANALYSIS

Remember, doing *something*—even if it fails—is better than doing nothing. You're gathering information.

Check in with the Body Mechanics Action Plans in Fix the Fire Damage for graduated activity recommendations that you can try safely and for immediate action. Use the companion manual, *Fix Your Body Mechanics* to strategize and track your progress.

What I have tried:

_____

_____

_____

_____

_____

_____

_____

_____

_____

What has worked:

_____

_____

_____

_____

_____

_____

_____

_____

What has *not* worked:

_____

_____

_____

_____

_____

_____

_____

_____

My
Coping
Journal

Overanalysis

MY COPING JOURNAL: OVERANALYSIS

_____

_____

_____

_____

_____

_____

_____

_____

_____

_____

_____

_____

_____

_____

_____

_____

_____

_____

_____

_____

_____

_____

_____

_____

_____

_____

_____

_____

_____

_____

_____

MY COPING JOURNAL: OVERANALYSIS

RELEASE UNCHECKED VENTING

Use these next several pages for some expressive writing. You may use the prompts but don't have to. (For more detailed guidance, refer to *Expressive Writing: Words that Heal* by James W. Pennebaker PhD. & John F. Evans.)

When this pain started, what happened and how did you feel both physically and emotionally?

_____

_____

_____

_____

_____

_____

_____

_____

_____

RELEASE UNCHECKED VENTING

What do you wish others understood about your experience with this pain?

_____

_____

_____

_____

_____

_____

_____

_____

_____

_____

_____

_____

_____

_____

_____

RELEASE UNCHECKED VENTING

Write a letter to yourself from your future pain-free self:

_____

_____

_____

_____

_____

_____

_____

_____

_____

_____

_____

_____

_____

_____

_____

RELEASE UNCHECKED VENTING

_____

_____

_____

_____

_____

_____

_____

_____

_____

_____

_____

_____

_____

My Coping Journal

Unchecked Venting

MY COPING JOURNAL: UNCHECKED VENTING

_____

_____

_____

_____

_____

_____

_____

_____

_____

_____

_____

_____

_____

_____

_____

_____

_____

_____

_____

_____

_____

_____

_____

_____

_____

_____

_____

_____

_____

MY COPING JOURNAL: UNCHECKED VENTING

_____

_____

_____

_____

_____

_____

_____

_____

_____

_____

_____

_____

_____

_____

_____

_____

THE FIVE S'S

A Remedy for All Four Coping Pitfalls

Most likely, we are all using a little bit of each of the four coping methods even if not all at the same time.

There is a pain coping self-coaching strategy that has emerged through the creation of this *Everyday Pain Guide* and it is the Five S's of Better Pain Coping. The Five S's were designed by Dr. Liou with pain in mind but can be applied for less toxicity inside of any and all four coping styles outlined above.

1. See It – pay attention to even the earliest signs of pain

2. Support It – validate your experience of pain

3. Specify – name it/find ways to describe it and give voice to it

4. Study It – be curious and open to its origin

5. Strategize – problem solve

You can start strategizing and problem solving right away with this book series but number 5 is ultimately something to be done with the help of a professional if necessary and armed with the first four S's, you can better set yourself up for a successful therapeutic experience with your provider of choice.

Think about how you talk to yourself at the onset of pain.

Are you telling yourself to suck it up and walk it off? Are you telling yourself it's hopeless and you deserve to be in pain because of something you did?

_____

_____

_____

_____

_____

_____

_____

_____

_____

_____

_____

THE FIVE S'S

Consider how you would talk to a tender young child.

What would you want to say to them if they were in the same situation? How can you let them know that you see them and their pain? How would you comfort them?

_____

_____

_____

_____

_____

_____

_____

_____

_____

_____

_____

_____

Consider how you see others' perceptions.

Are you distracted by thoughts of how others will see you or what
they will say once you reveal that you have pain? Whose voices are
those?

_____

_____

_____

_____

_____

_____

_____

_____

_____

_____

_____

_____

THE FIVE S'S

How can you reframe things to provide the support of The Five S's that others in your life may not be able to give you?

Try saying these following things out loud to yourself:

"I did nothing wrong."

"My body is giving me important information."

"I feel _____ (frustrated/scared/angry…) and that's okay."

"I'm curious to learn what my body wants me to know."

Create your own mantra(s) to help support The Five S's.

_____

_____

_____

_____

_____

_____

_____

_____

How did saying these things out loud make you feel?

_____

_____

_____

_____

_____

_____

Is there something else that you want to say to yourself?

_____

_____

_____

_____

_____

_____

THE FIVE S'S

I would describe my pain like this:
(Use descriptive words like "aching", "stabbing", "sharp", "dull", "tingling", "grabbing" etc.)

_____

_____

_____

_____

_____

_____

_____

_____

_____

_____

_____

_____

_____

My pain reminds me of:

(Think of other sensation or experiences you've had in the past or think of a time in your life and the details of those circumstances - no matter how unrelated they might seem to you right now.)

_____

_____

_____

_____

_____

_____

_____

_____

_____

_____

_____

_____

_____

_____

My Coping Journal

The Five S's

_____

_____

_____

_____

_____

_____

_____

_____

_____

_____

_____

_____

_____

_____

_____

_____

THE FIVE S'S

_____

_____

_____

_____

_____

_____

_____

_____

_____

_____

_____

_____

_____

_____

_____

_____

_____

_____

_____

_____

_____

_____

_____

_____

_____

_____

_____

_____

_____

_____

_____

RETRAIN YOUR NERVOUS SYSTEM USING YOUR FIVE SENSES

What scents do you remember from childhood or carefree younger years?

_____

_____

_____

_____

_____

_____

_____

_____

_____

_____

_____

What scents make you happy?

_____

_____

_____

_____

_____

_____

_____

_____

_____

_____

_____

_____

_____

_____

RETRAIN YOUR NERVOUS SYSTEM

Do you have a favorite slippers, pajamas, blankets, or a hat? What makes those items soothing for you? How can you bring that same element to more parts of your day?

_____

_____

_____

_____

_____

_____

_____

_____

_____

_____

_____

_____

_____

Does heat feel soothing for you? What sounds best to you: a bath, a sauna, a heating pad, or a warming menthol lotion? Try one and take note of how it affects your pain:

_____

_____

_____

_____

_____

_____

_____

_____

_____

_____

_____

_____

_____

_____

Does ice feel nice or annoying? What happens when you apply an ice pack? What if you apply heat somewhere else on your body at the same time as ice to your pain?

_____

_____

_____

_____

_____

_____

_____

_____

_____

_____

_____

_____

_____

Have you tried receiving a massage or any other touch therapy? Do you enjoy vigorous deep touch? Do you prefer a gentle light touch? How does your body feel after each type of touch?

_____

_____

_____

_____

_____

_____

_____

_____

_____

_____

_____

_____

_____

_____

Do you find firm pressure soothing? Do you like your bed sheets firmly tucked? Maybe you would enjoy a weighted blanket?

_____

_____

_____

_____

_____

_____

_____

_____

_____

_____

_____

_____

_____

_____

What sort of sounds bring you joy? Do you remember a song from your youth that makes you want to dance? Maybe there's a theme song from a movie that transports you to a magical place in your mind? Is there a particular instrument that gives you pleasant goosebumps to listen to? Jot down some ideas:

_____

_____

_____

_____

_____

_____

_____

_____

_____

_____

_____

_____

_____

RETRAIN YOUR NERVOUS SYSTEM

How often do you have the opportunity to gaze into the distance at the treetops or into the clouds or across town from a balcony on the 34th floor? Make a plan for when you can use panoramic vision in your day and savor it. How does it make you feel just to imagine it? Do you notice your shoulders dropping?

_____

_____

_____

_____

_____

_____

_____

_____

_____

_____

_____

_____

RETRAIN YOUR GLUCOSE METABOLISM

Food

Please return to the Body Chemistry Action Plan in Section II of *Fix the Fire Damage* and use the companion manual *Fix Your Body Chemistry* for guidance about navigating a strategic pause from the Big Three garbage items.

My Food:

Do I have social or emotional barriers to taking a break from the Big Three? What are they?

_____

_____

_____

_____

_____

_____

_____

_____

My Food:

Do I have social and emotional support for taking a break from the Big Three? How can I nurture this support?

_____

_____

_____

_____

_____

_____

_____

_____

_____

_____

_____

_____

_____

_____

_____

_____

Retrain Your Glucose Metabolism Journal

Food

RETRAIN YOUR GLUCOSE METABOLISM: FOOD

_____

_____

_____

_____

_____

_____

_____

_____

_____

_____

_____

_____

_____

_____

_____

Retrain Your Glucose Metabolism Journal

My Sleep Diary

TODAY'S DATE: _____

Bedtime:

_____

Wakeup time:

_____

**Number of toilet
breaks or significant
wakeups in the night:**

_____

Total hours of rest:

_____

Last night's meal:

What time was my last meal last night? _____

What did I eat?

_____

_____

First meal this morning:

What time was my first meal this morning? _____

What did I eat?

_____

_____

How is my mood today?

_____

_____

_____

_____

_____

_____

What else happened today that influenced my food choices, my mood, my bedtime and waketime?

_____

_____

_____

_____

_____

_____

TODAY'S DATE: _____

Bedtime:
_____

Wakeup time:
_____

**Number of toilet
breaks or significant
wakeups in the night:**
_____

Total hours of rest:
_____

Last night's meal:

What time was my last meal last night? _____

What did I eat?

_____

_____

First meal this morning:

What time was my first meal this morning? _____

What did I eat?

_____

_____

How is my mood today?

_____

_____

_____

_____

_____

_____

What else happened today that influenced my food choices, my mood, my bedtime and waketime?

_____

_____

_____

_____

_____

_____

TODAY'S DATE: _____

Bedtime: _____

Wakeup time: _____

Number of toilet breaks or significant wakeups in the night: _____

Total hours of rest: _____

Last night's meal:

What time was my last meal last night? _____

What did I eat?

_____

_____

First meal this morning:

What time was my first meal this morning? _____

What did I eat?

_____

_____

How is my mood today?

_____

_____

_____

_____

_____

_____

What else happened today that influenced my food choices, my mood, my bedtime and waketime?

_____

_____

_____

_____

_____

_____

_____

TODAY'S DATE: _____

Bedtime: _____

Wakeup time: _____

Number of toilet breaks or significant wakeups in the night: _____

Total hours of rest: _____

Last night's meal:

What time was my last meal last night? _____

What did I eat?

_____

_____

First meal this morning:

What time was my first meal this morning? _____

What did I eat?

_____

_____

How is my mood today?

_____

_____

_____

_____

_____

_____

What else happened today that influenced my food choices, my mood, my bedtime and waketime?

_____

_____

_____

_____

_____

_____

_____

TODAY'S DATE:

Bedtime:

Wakeup time:

**Number of toilet
breaks or significant
wakeups in the night:**

Total hours of rest:

Last night's meal:

What time was my last meal last night? _____

What did I eat?

_____

_____

First meal this morning:

What time was my first meal this morning? _____

What did I eat?

_____

_____

How is my mood today?

_____

_____

_____

_____

_____

What else happened today that influenced my food choices, my mood, my bedtime and waketime?

_____

_____

_____

_____

_____

TODAY'S DATE: _____

    Bedtime:

_____

    Wakeup time:

_____

    Number of toilet
    breaks or significant
    wakeups in the night:

_____

    Total hours of rest:

_____

Last night's meal:

What time was my last meal last night? _____

What did I eat?

_____

_____

First meal this morning:

What time was my first meal this morning? _____

What did I eat?

_____

_____

How is my mood today?

_____

_____

_____

_____

_____

_____

What else happened today that influenced my food choices, my mood, my bedtime and waketime?

_____

_____

_____

_____

_____

_____

TODAY'S DATE: _____

Bedtime: _____

Wakeup time: _____

Number of toilet breaks or significant wakeups in the night: _____

Total hours of rest: _____

Last night's meal:

What time was my last meal last night? _____

What did I eat?

_____

_____

First meal this morning:

What time was my first meal this morning? _____

What did I eat?

_____

_____

How is my mood today?

_____

_____

_____

_____

_____

_____

What else happened today that influenced my food choices, my mood, my bedtime and waketime?

_____

_____

_____

_____

_____

_____

RETRAIN YOUR
GLUCOSE METABOLISM

PLAY

What's my version of play?

_____

_____

_____

_____

_____

_____

_____

_____

_____

_____

What do I look forward to after work or school, in the evenings or on weekends?

(Suggestions: team sports/gym workouts/kids/pets/watching others etc.)

_____

_____

_____

_____

_____

Do I want to be playful more often?

Circle one: Yes / No

Details:_____

_____

_____

Who can I play with?

_____

_____

_____

_____

Retrain Your Glucose Metabolism Journal

Play

_____

_____

_____

_____

_____

_____

_____

_____

_____

_____

_____

_____

_____

_____

_____

_____

_____

_____

_____

_____

_____

_____

_____

_____

_____

_____

_____

_____

_____

_____

_____

RETRAIN YOUR GLUCOSE METABOLISM

RELATIONSHIPS

Work:

Who do I feel stressed around when I'm at work?

_____

_____

_____

_____

_____

_____

_____

_____

_____

RETRAIN YOUR GLUCOSE METABOLISM: RELATIONSHIPS

Is it possible to spend less time with this person?

Circle one: Yes / No

If not, what are some ideas for how I can change my response to that person:

_____

_____

_____

_____

_____

_____

_____

_____

_____

_____

_____

_____

Home:

Who do I feel stressed around when I'm at home?

_____

_____

_____

_____

_____

_____

_____

_____

_____

_____

_____

_____

_____

RETRAIN YOUR GLUCOSE METABOLISM: RELATIONSHIPS

Is it possible to spend less time with this person?

Circle one: Yes / No

If not, what are some ideas for how I can change my response to that person:

_____

_____

_____

_____

_____

_____

_____

_____

_____

_____

_____

_____

Friends/Other:

Who do I feel stressed around in my friend or social group?

_____

_____

_____

_____

_____

_____

_____

_____

_____

_____

_____

_____

_____

RETRAIN YOUR GLUCOSE METABOLISM: RELATIONSHIPS

Is it possible to spend less time with this person?

Circle one: Yes / No

If not, what are some ideas for how I can change my response to that person:

_____

_____

_____

_____

_____

_____

_____

_____

_____

_____

_____

_____

Please consider seeking professional guidance from a therapist or a counselor to help you answer some of these questions about relationships.

If you don't feel safe, please consider your local crisis hotline or dialing 988 for the national crisis line.

Retrain Your Glucose Metabolism Journal

Relationships

_____

_____

_____

_____

_____

_____

_____

_____

_____

_____

_____

_____

_____

_____

_____

RELEASE FEAR POSTURES

by Retraining Safety Postures

Think of what you can do to remind your body (and nervous system) that you don't have to be in this shape—physically or emotionally.

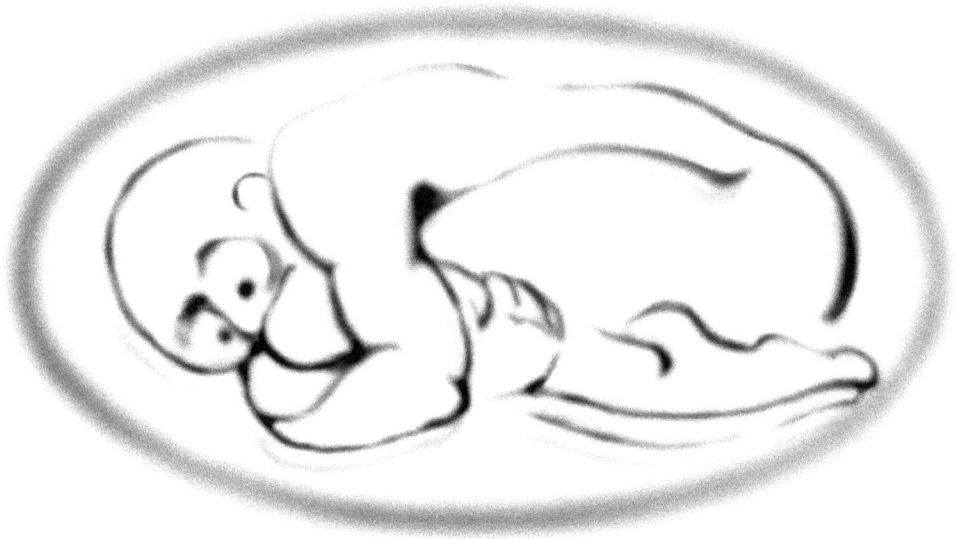

_____

_____

_____

_____

_____

_____

_____

_____

_____

_____

_____

_____

_____

_____

_____

RELEASE FEAR POSTURES

Refer to the Body Mechanics Action Plans for ideas on how to activate the muscles that hold your body more like this:

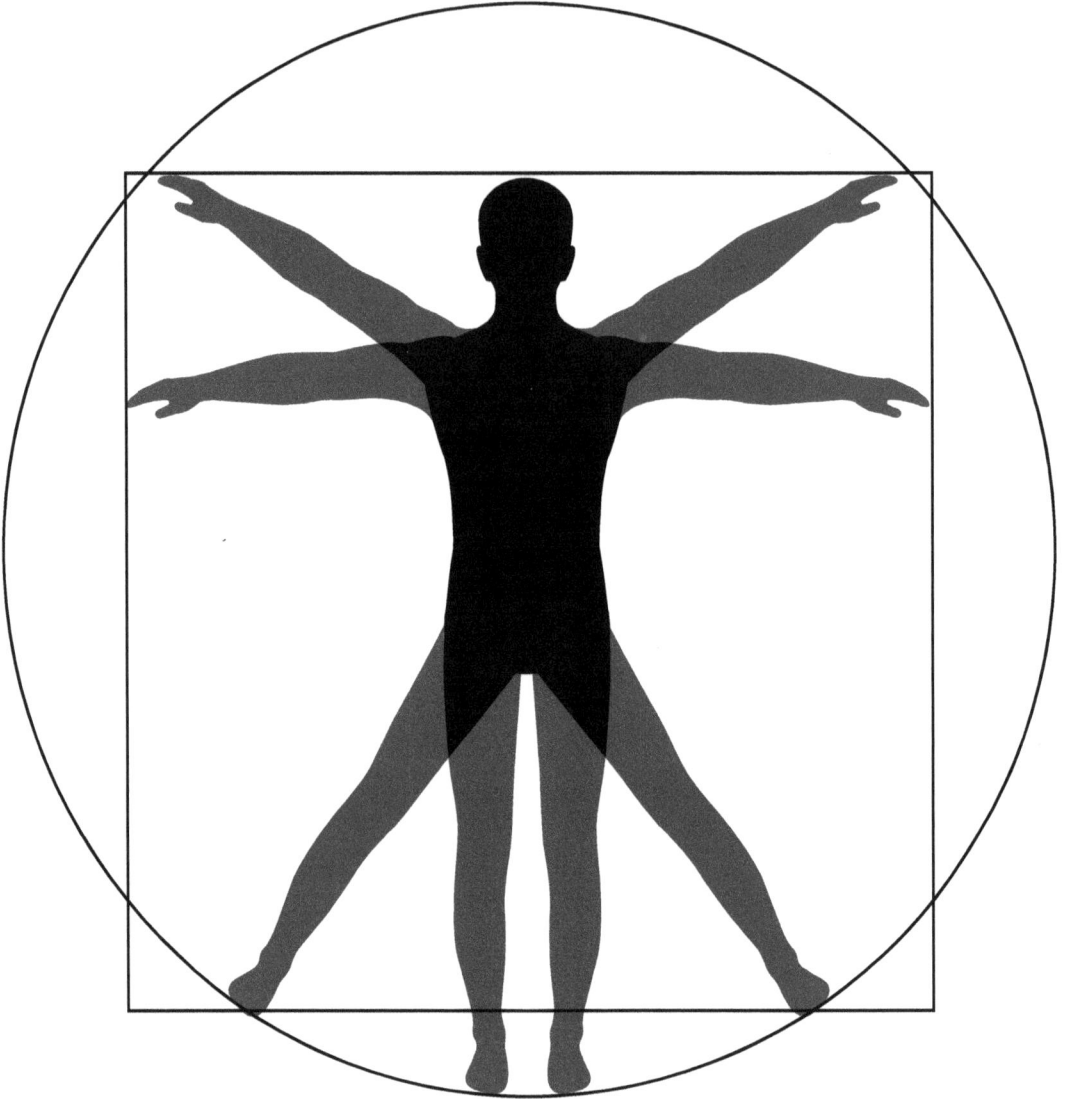

Think of all the times during a routine day when your body is not in its most open position. Consider how you can adopt more open and vulnerable body positioning. How do you feel when you do this?

_____

_____

_____

_____

_____

_____

_____

_____

_____

_____

_____

_____

_____

_____

As the saying goes:

"Don't believe

everything

you think."

RETRAIN YOUR HEALTH AND WELLNESS BIASES

Consider the following affirmations.

Say them out loud.

Write down and sketch your thoughts.

Modify them to make your own.

AFFIRMATION:

Pain and suffering are not an inevitable part of aging.

My Thoughts:

_____

_____

_____

_____

_____

_____

_____

RETRAIN YOUR HEALTH AND WELLNESS BIASES

My Thoughts:

AFFIRMATION:

People of all sizes can have pain and many plus sized people do not have pain.

My Thoughts:

_____

_____

_____

_____

_____

_____

_____

RETRAIN YOUR HEALTH AND WELLNESS BIASES

My Thoughts:

AFFIRMATION:

My body is shaped the way it is for a reason.

My Thoughts:

_____

_____

_____

_____

_____

_____

_____

RETRAIN YOUR HEALTH AND WELLNESS BIASES

My Thoughts:

AFFIRMATION:

The human body is inherently asymmetrical. Aspiring to be symmetrical will not necessarily solve my pain problem.

My Thoughts:

_____

_____

_____

_____

My Thoughts:

AFFIRMATION:

My body is making genius adaptations every day.

My Thoughts:

_____

_____

_____

_____

_____

_____

_____

RETRAIN YOUR HEALTH AND WELLNESS BIASES

My Thoughts:

AFFIRMATION:

I trust my body.

My Thoughts:

_____

_____

_____

_____

_____

_____

_____

_____

My Thoughts:

AFFIRMATIONS

Consider what your own affirmations are. Write them down or sketch out some ideas.

_____

_____

_____

_____

_____

_____

_____

_____

_____

_____

_____

RETRAIN YOUR HEALTH AND WELLNESS BIASES

AFFIRMATIONS

Consider what your own affirmations are. Write them down or sketch out some ideas.

_____

_____

_____

_____

_____

_____

_____

_____

_____

_____

_____

_____

RETRAIN YOUR HEALTH AND WELLNESS BIASES

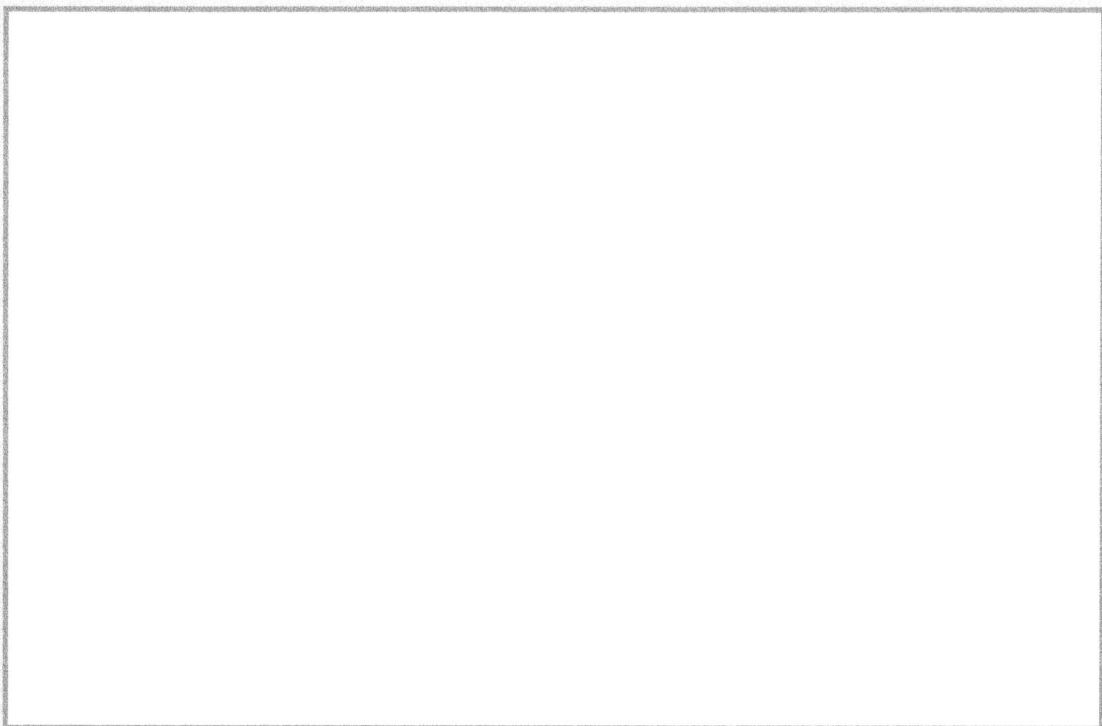

My *Reinforce* Action Steps

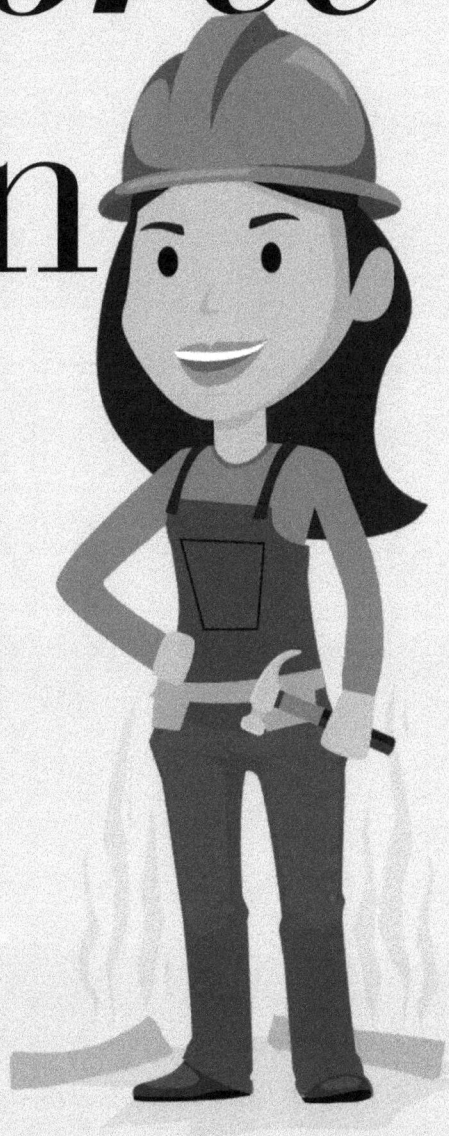

THE CHECK IN

How are you feeling?

TODAY'S DATE: _____

PAIN LOCATION:
(circle one)

Neck   Neck/Shoulder   Shoulder/Upper Back   Mid Back/Torso/Ribs

Low Back   Low Back/Hip   Hip/Buttock/Thigh

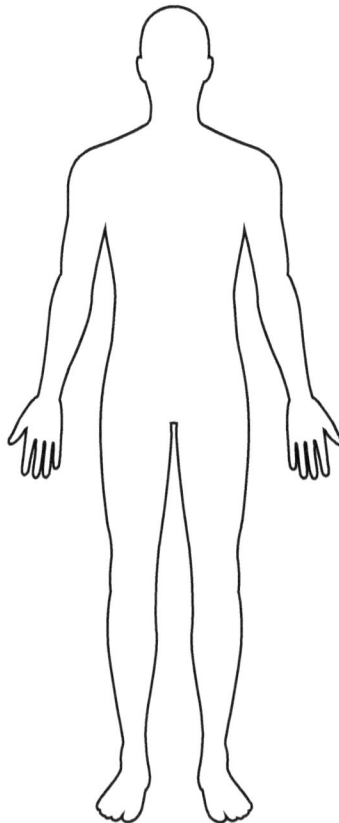

Use this figure to color or shade-in the area of your pain however you like.

HOW MUCH PAIN TODAY?

Circle the face below that best expresses your discomfort:

Wong-Baker FACES® Pain Rating Scale

0	2	4	6	8	10
No Pain	A Little Pain	A Little More Pain	Even More Pain	A Whole Lot Of Pain	Worst Pain

Notes:

_____

_____

_____

_____

_____

_____

_____

_____

_____

REINFORCE!

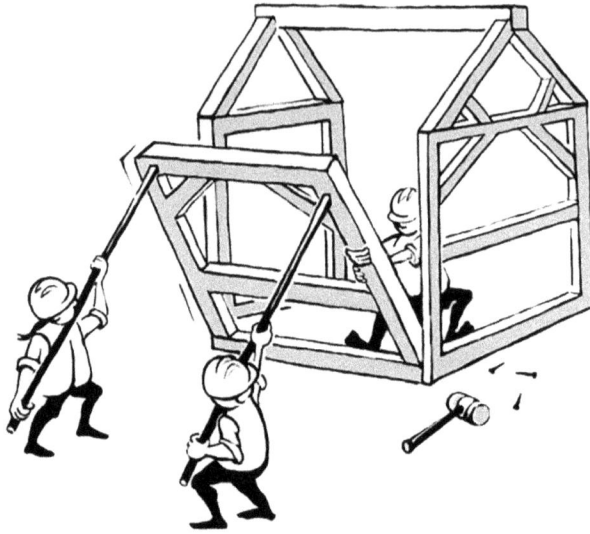

Q: *What* is being reinforced?

A: **Your low-stress biology**

Q: *How* will your low-stress biology be reinforced?

A: **By easing up on yourself, keeping it up and returning to it**

➤ Go to the book for more: *Fix the Fire Damage*, pages 512 - 513

➤ Listen to the podcast: *Conversations About Everyday Pain*, Season 2, Episodes 582

NEXT STEPS:

1.   Ease up on yourself

2.   Keep it up

3.   Return to your self-care when you stray

SELF-CARE:

Real self-care is a practice not a treat or a reward.

*The reward from such dedicated self-care is a life
with less inflammatory stress in your body.*

When we teach others what we've learned, it helps us reinforce and better integrate new information in our own lives. Find someone with whom you can share insights from your Everyday Pain Guide journey.

MY SELF-CARE PRACTICE

What activities and/or responsibilities drain my energy or do *not* bring joy?

☐ _____

☐ _____

☐ _____

☐ _____

☐ _____

☐ _____

☐ _____

☐ _____

☐ _____

☐ _____

My obstacles to practicing self-care are...

☐ _____

☐ _____

☐ _____

☐ _____

☐ _____

☐ _____

☐ _____

☐ _____

☐ _____

☐ _____

☐ _____

☐ _____

MY SELF-CARE PRACTICE

What are some activities that bring joy and happiness? List as many as you can think of below.

☐ _____

☐ _____

☐ _____

☐ _____

☐ _____

☐ _____

☐ _____

☐ _____

☐ _____

☐ _____

☐ _____

☐ _____

Am I taking enough time to relax?

Circle one: Yes / No

Details:_____

_____

_____

_____

What are the things that inspire me?

_____

_____

_____

_____

_____

_____

_____

_____

_____

MY SELF-CARE PRACTICE

My goals for practicing self-care are...

☐ _____

☐ _____

☐ _____

☐ _____

☐ _____

☐ _____

☐ _____

☐ _____

☐ _____

☐ _____

☐ _____

☐ _____

My Self-Care Journal

TODAY'S DATE: _____

My goal(s) for today: I am grateful for...

_____   1. _____

_____   2. _____

_____   3. _____

_____   4. _____

_____   5. _____

How I feel today:
(mark with an X)

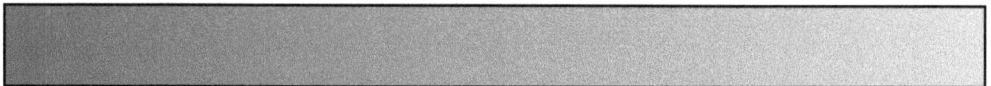

SAD   HAPPY

_____

_____

_____

_____

_____

IDEAS:

- play
- sleep
- social time
- quiet time
- spa/facial/massage etc.
- walk in nature
- daydreaming
- cook for myself
- order in

Self-Care Activity For Today

IDEAS:

- Taking care of myself gives me more to share with others.
- It is kind and wise to honor my limits.
- I allow myself to feel without judgment and release what no longer serves me.
- My thoughts can soften; I can choose peace in this moment.
- It is safe for me to slow down, breathe, and simply be.
- I give my body what it needs to feel nourished and supported.
- I listen with respect to the messages my body sends me.
- Rest is productive; my body heals and restores when I pause.

Today's Affirmation

TODAY'S DATE: _____

My goal(s) for today: I am grateful for...

_____   1. _____

_____   2. _____

_____   3. _____

_____   4. _____

_____   5. _____

How I feel today:
(mark with an X)

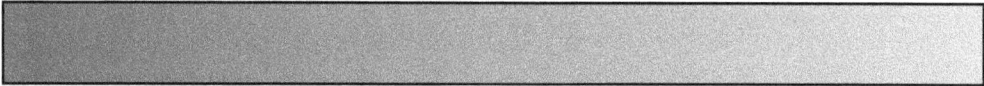

SAD   HAPPY

_____

_____

_____

_____

_____

IDEAS:

- play
- sleep
- social time
- quiet time
- spa/facial/massage etc.
- walk in nature
- daydreaming
- cook for myself
- order in

Self-Care Activity For Today

IDEAS:

- Taking care of myself gives me more to share with others.
- It is kind and wise to honor my limits.
- I allow myself to feel without judgment and release what no longer serves me.
- My thoughts can soften; I can choose peace in this moment.
- It is safe for me to slow down, breathe, and simply be.
- I give my body what it needs to feel nourished and supported.
- I listen with respect to the messages my body sends me.
- Rest is productive; my body heals and restores when I pause.

Today's Affirmation

TODAY'S DATE: _____

My goal(s) for today: I am grateful for...

_____   1. _____

_____   2. _____

_____   3. _____

_____   4. _____

_____   5. _____

How I feel today:
(mark with an X)

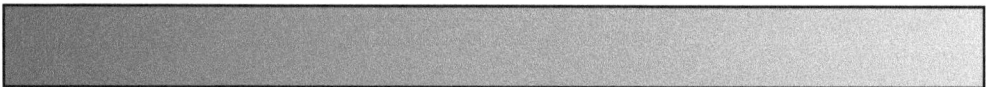

SAD   HAPPY

_____

_____

_____

_____

_____

IDEAS:

- play
- sleep
- social time
- quiet time
- spa/facial/massage etc.
- walk in nature
- daydreaming
- cook for myself
- order in

Self-Care Activity For Today

IDEAS:

- Taking care of myself gives me more to share with others.
- It is kind and wise to honor my limits.
- I allow myself to feel without judgment and release what no longer serves me.
- My thoughts can soften; I can choose peace in this moment.
- It is safe for me to slow down, breathe, and simply be.
- I give my body what it needs to feel nourished and supported.
- I listen with respect to the messages my body sends me.
- Rest is productive; my body heals and restores when I pause.

Today's Affirmation

TODAY'S DATE: _____

My goal(s) for today: I am grateful for...

_____   1. _____

_____   2. _____

_____   3. _____

_____   4. _____

_____   5. _____

How I feel today:
(mark with an X)

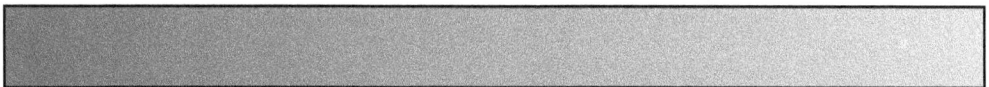

SAD   HAPPY

_____

_____

_____

_____

_____

Self-Care Activity For Today

IDEAS:

- play
- sleep
- social time
- quiet time
- spa/facial/massage etc.
- walk in nature
- daydreaming
- cook for myself
- order in

Today's Affirmation

IDEAS:

- Taking care of myself gives me more to share with others.
- It is kind and wise to honor my limits.
- I allow myself to feel without judgment and release what no longer serves me.
- My thoughts can soften; I can choose peace in this moment.
- It is safe for me to slow down, breathe, and simply be.
- I give my body what it needs to feel nourished and supported.
- I listen with respect to the messages my body sends me.
- Rest is productive; my body heals and restores when I pause.

TODAY'S DATE: _____

My goal(s) for today: I am grateful for...

_____   1. _____

_____   2. _____

_____   3. _____

_____   4. _____

_____   5. _____

How I feel today:
(mark with an X)

SAD   HAPPY

_____

_____

_____

_____

_____

Self-Care Activity For Today

IDEAS:

- play
- sleep
- social time
- quiet time
- spa/facial/massage etc.
- walk in nature
- daydreaming
- cook for myself
- order in

Today's Affirmation

IDEAS:

- Taking care of myself gives me more to share with others.
- It is kind and wise to honor my limits.
- I allow myself to feel without judgment and release what no longer serves me.
- My thoughts can soften; I can choose peace in this moment.
- It is safe for me to slow down, breathe, and simply be.
- I give my body what it needs to feel nourished and supported.
- I listen with respect to the messages my body sends me.
- Rest is productive; my body heals and restores when I pause.

TODAY'S DATE: _____

My goal(s) for today: I am grateful for...

_____   1. _____

_____   2. _____

_____   3. _____

_____   4. _____

_____   5. _____

How I feel today:
(mark with an X)

SAD   HAPPY

_____

_____

_____

_____

_____

Self-Care Activity For Today

IDEAS:

- play
- sleep
- social time
- quiet time
- spa/facial/massage etc.
- walk in nature
- daydreaming
- cook for myself
- order in

Today's Affirmation

IDEAS:

- Taking care of myself gives me more to share with others.
- It is kind and wise to honor my limits.
- I allow myself to feel without judgment and release what no longer serves me.
- My thoughts can soften; I can choose peace in this moment.
- It is safe for me to slow down, breathe, and simply be.
- I give my body what it needs to feel nourished and supported.
- I listen with respect to the messages my body sends me.
- Rest is productive; my body heals and restores when I pause.

TODAY'S DATE: _____

My goal(s) for today: I am grateful for...

_____   1. _____

_____   2. _____

_____   3. _____

_____   4. _____

_____   5. _____

How I feel today:
(mark with an X)

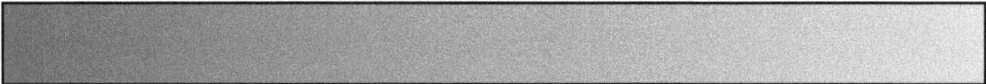

SAD   HAPPY

_____

_____

_____

_____

_____

_____

Self-Care Activity For Today

IDEAS:

➤ play
➤ sleep
➤ social time
➤ quiet time
➤ spa/facial/massage etc.
➤ walk in nature
➤ daydreaming
➤ cook for myself
➤ order in

Today's Affirmation

IDEAS:

➤ Taking care of myself gives me more to share with others.
➤ It is kind and wise to honor my limits.
➤ I allow myself to feel without judgment and release what no longer serves me.
➤ My thoughts can soften; I can choose peace in this moment.
➤ It is safe for me to slow down, breathe, and simply be.
➤ I give my body what it needs to feel nourished and supported.
➤ I listen with respect to the messages my body sends me.
➤ Rest is productive; my body heals and restores when I pause.

TODAY'S DATE: _____

My goal(s) for today:

I am grateful for...

_____

1. _____

_____

2. _____

_____

3. _____

_____

4. _____

_____

5. _____

How I feel today:
(mark with an X)

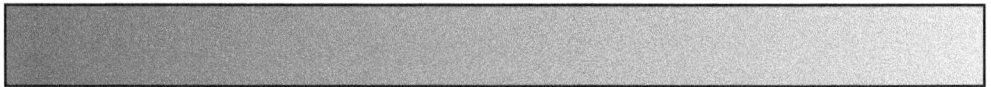

SAD   HAPPY

_____

_____

_____

_____

_____

Self-Care Activity For Today

IDEAS:

- play
- sleep
- social time
- quiet time
- spa/facial/massage etc.
- walk in nature
- daydreaming
- cook for myself
- order in

Today's Affirmation

IDEAS:

- Taking care of myself gives me more to share with others.
- It is kind and wise to honor my limits.
- I allow myself to feel without judgment and release what no longer serves me.
- My thoughts can soften; I can choose peace in this moment.
- It is safe for me to slow down, breathe, and simply be.
- I give my body what it needs to feel nourished and supported.
- I listen with respect to the messages my body sends me.
- Rest is productive; my body heals and restores when I pause.

TODAY'S DATE: _____

My goal(s) for today: I am grateful for...

_____   1. _____

_____   2. _____

_____   3. _____

_____   4. _____

_____   5. _____

How I feel today:
(mark with an X)

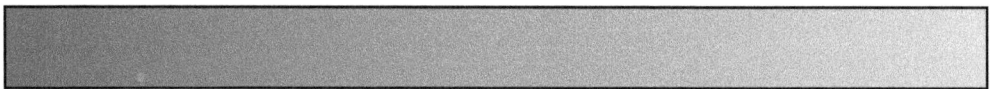

SAD   HAPPY

_____

_____

_____

_____

_____

_____

Self-Care Activity For Today

IDEAS:

- ➤ play
- ➤ sleep
- ➤ social time
- ➤ quiet time
- ➤ spa/facial/massage etc.
- ➤ walk in nature
- ➤ daydreaming
- ➤ cook for myself
- ➤ order in

Today's Affirmation

IDEAS:

- ➤ Taking care of myself gives me more to share with others.
- ➤ It is kind and wise to honor my limits.
- ➤ I allow myself to feel without judgment and release what no longer serves me.
- ➤ My thoughts can soften; I can choose peace in this moment.
- ➤ It is safe for me to slow down, breathe, and simply be.
- ➤ I give my body what it needs to feel nourished and supported.
- ➤ I listen with respect to the messages my body sends me.
- ➤ Rest is productive; my body heals and restores when I pause.

TODAY'S DATE: _____

My goal(s) for today:

_____

_____

_____

_____

_____

I am grateful for...

1. _____

2. _____

3. _____

4. _____

5. _____

How I feel today:
(mark with an X)

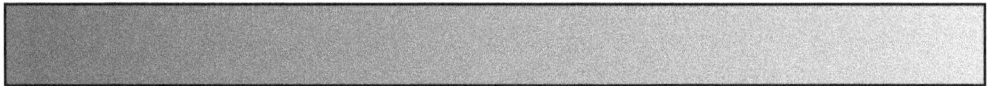

SAD   HAPPY

_____

_____

_____

_____

_____

IDEAS:

- play
- sleep
- social time
- quiet time
- spa/facial/massage etc.
- walk in nature
- daydreaming
- cook for myself
- order in

Self-Care Activity For Today

IDEAS:

- Taking care of myself gives me more to share with others.
- It is kind and wise to honor my limits.
- I allow myself to feel without judgment and release what no longer serves me.
- My thoughts can soften; I can choose peace in this moment.
- It is safe for me to slow down, breathe, and simply be.
- I give my body what it needs to feel nourished and supported.
- I listen with respect to the messages my body sends me.
- Rest is productive; my body heals and restores when I pause.

Today's Affirmation

TODAY'S DATE: _____

My goal(s) for today: I am grateful for...

_____   1. _____

_____   2. _____

_____   3. _____

_____   4. _____

_____   5. _____

How I feel today:
(mark with an X)

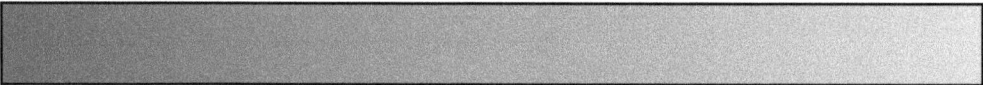

SAD   HAPPY

_____

_____

_____

_____

_____

_____

IDEAS:

➤ play
➤ sleep
➤ social time
➤ quiet time
➤ spa/facial/massage etc.
➤ walk in nature
➤ daydreaming
➤ cook for myself
➤ order in

Self-Care Activity For Today

IDEAS:

➤ Taking care of myself gives me more to share with others.
➤ It is kind and wise to honor my limits.
➤ I allow myself to feel without judgment and release what no longer serves me.
➤ My thoughts can soften; I can choose peace in this moment.
➤ It is safe for me to slow down, breathe, and simply be.
➤ I give my body what it needs to feel nourished and supported.
➤ I listen with respect to the messages my body sends me.
➤ Rest is productive; my body heals and restores when I pause.

Today's Affirmation

TODAY'S DATE: _____

My goal(s) for today: I am grateful for...

_____   1. _____

_____   2. _____

_____   3. _____

_____   4. _____

_____   5. _____

How I feel today:
(mark with an X)

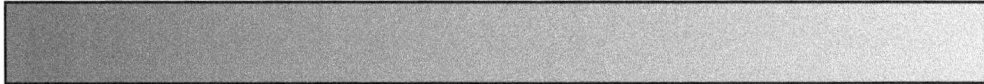

SAD   HAPPY

_____

_____

_____

_____

_____

IDEAS:

- play
- sleep
- social time
- quiet time
- spa/facial/massage etc.
- walk in nature
- daydreaming
- cook for myself
- order in

Self-Care Activity For Today

IDEAS:

- Taking care of myself gives me more to share with others.
- It is kind and wise to honor my limits.
- I allow myself to feel without judgment and release what no longer serves me.
- My thoughts can soften; I can choose peace in this moment.
- It is safe for me to slow down, breathe, and simply be.
- I give my body what it needs to feel nourished and supported.
- I listen with respect to the messages my body sends me.
- Rest is productive; my body heals and restores when I pause.

Today's Affirmation

TODAY'S DATE: _____

My goal(s) for today: I am grateful for...

_____   1. _____

_____   2. _____

_____   3. _____

_____   4. _____

_____   5. _____

How I feel today:
(mark with an X)

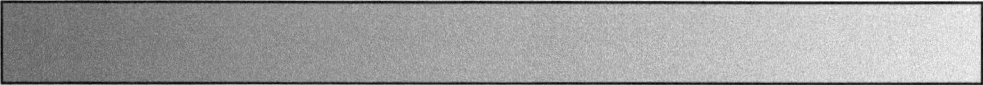

SAD   HAPPY

_____

_____

_____

_____

_____

IDEAS:

- play
- sleep
- social time
- quiet time
- spa/facial/massage etc.
- walk in nature
- daydreaming
- cook for myself
- order in

Self-Care Activity For Today

IDEAS:

- Taking care of myself gives me more to share with others.
- It is kind and wise to honor my limits.
- I allow myself to feel without judgment and release what no longer serves me.
- My thoughts can soften; I can choose peace in this moment.
- It is safe for me to slow down, breathe, and simply be.
- I give my body what it needs to feel nourished and supported.
- I listen with respect to the messages my body sends me.
- Rest is productive; my body heals and restores when I pause.

Today's Affirmation

TODAY'S DATE: _____

My goal(s) for today: I am grateful for...

_____   1. _____

_____   2. _____

_____   3. _____

_____   4. _____

_____   5. _____

How I feel today:
(mark with an X)

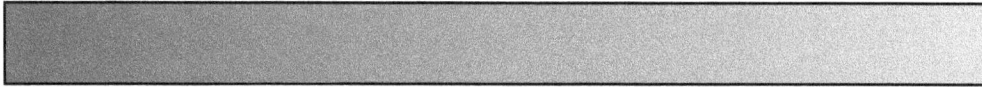

SAD   HAPPY

_____

_____

_____

_____

_____

_____

IDEAS:

- play
- sleep
- social time
- quiet time
- spa/facial/massage etc.
- walk in nature
- daydreaming
- cook for myself
- order in

Self-Care Activity For Today

IDEAS:

- Taking care of myself gives me more to share with others.
- It is kind and wise to honor my limits.
- I allow myself to feel without judgment and release what no longer serves me.
- My thoughts can soften; I can choose peace in this moment.
- It is safe for me to slow down, breathe, and simply be.
- I give my body what it needs to feel nourished and supported.
- I listen with respect to the messages my body sends me.
- Rest is productive; my body heals and restores when I pause.

Today's Affirmation

TODAY'S DATE: _____

My goal(s) for today:

_____

_____

_____

_____

_____

I am grateful for...

1. _____

2. _____

3. _____

4. _____

5. _____

How I feel today:
(mark with an X)

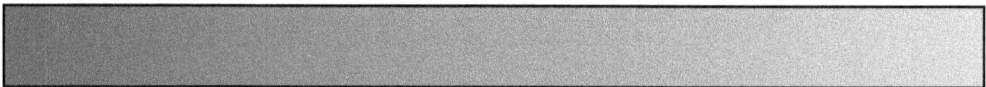

SAD   HAPPY

_____

_____

_____

_____

_____

IDEAS:

- ➤ play
- ➤ sleep
- ➤ social time
- ➤ quiet time
- ➤ spa/facial/massage etc.
- ➤ walk in nature
- ➤ daydreaming
- ➤ cook for myself
- ➤ order in

Self-Care Activity For Today

IDEAS:

- ➤ Taking care of myself gives me more to share with others.
- ➤ It is kind and wise to honor my limits.
- ➤ I allow myself to feel without judgment and release what no longer serves me.
- ➤ My thoughts can soften; I can choose peace in this moment.
- ➤ It is safe for me to slow down, breathe, and simply be.
- ➤ I give my body what it needs to feel nourished and supported.
- ➤ I listen with respect to the messages my body sends me.
- ➤ Rest is productive; my body heals and restores when I pause.

Today's Affirmation

TODAY'S DATE: _____

My goal(s) for today: I am grateful for...

_____   1. _____

_____   2. _____

_____   3. _____

_____   4. _____

_____   5. _____

How I feel today:
(mark with an X)

SAD   HAPPY

_____

_____

_____

_____

_____

Self-Care Activity For Today

IDEAS:

➤ play
➤ sleep
➤ social time
➤ quiet time
➤ spa/facial/massage etc.
➤ walk in nature
➤ daydreaming
➤ cook for myself
➤ order in

Today's Affirmation

IDEAS:

➤ Taking care of myself gives me more to share with others.
➤ It is kind and wise to honor my limits.
➤ I allow myself to feel without judgment and release what no longer serves me.
➤ My thoughts can soften; I can choose peace in this moment.
➤ It is safe for me to slow down, breathe, and simply be.
➤ I give my body what it needs to feel nourished and supported.
➤ I listen with respect to the messages my body sends me.
➤ Rest is productive; my body heals and restores when I pause.

TODAY'S DATE: _____

My goal(s) for today: I am grateful for...

_____   1. _____

_____   2. _____

_____   3. _____

_____   4. _____

_____   5. _____

How I feel today:
(mark with an X)

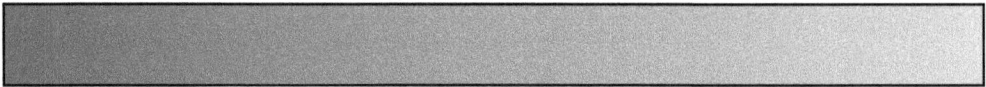

SAD   HAPPY

_____

_____

_____

_____

_____

IDEAS:

- play
- sleep
- social time
- quiet time
- spa/facial/massage etc.
- walk in nature
- daydreaming
- cook for myself
- order in

Self-Care Activity For Today

IDEAS:

- Taking care of myself gives me more to share with others.
- It is kind and wise to honor my limits.
- I allow myself to feel without judgment and release what no longer serves me.
- My thoughts can soften; I can choose peace in this moment.
- It is safe for me to slow down, breathe, and simply be.
- I give my body what it needs to feel nourished and supported.
- I listen with respect to the messages my body sends me.
- Rest is productive; my body heals and restores when I pause.

Today's Affirmation

TODAY'S DATE: _____

My goal(s) for today:

_____

_____

_____

_____

_____

I am grateful for...

1. _____

2. _____

3. _____

4. _____

5. _____

How I feel today:
(mark with an X)

SAD   HAPPY

_____

_____

_____

_____

_____

IDEAS:

- play
- sleep
- social time
- quiet time
- spa/facial/massage etc.
- walk in nature
- daydreaming
- cook for myself
- order in

Self-Care Activity For Today

IDEAS:

- Taking care of myself gives me more to share with others.
- It is kind and wise to honor my limits.
- I allow myself to feel without judgment and release what no longer serves me.
- My thoughts can soften; I can choose peace in this moment.
- It is safe for me to slow down, breathe, and simply be.
- I give my body what it needs to feel nourished and supported.
- I listen with respect to the messages my body sends me.
- Rest is productive; my body heals and restores when I pause.

Today's Affirmation

TODAY'S DATE: _____

My goal(s) for today: I am grateful for...

_____   1. _____

_____   2. _____

_____   3. _____

_____   4. _____

_____   5. _____

How I feel today:
(mark with an X)

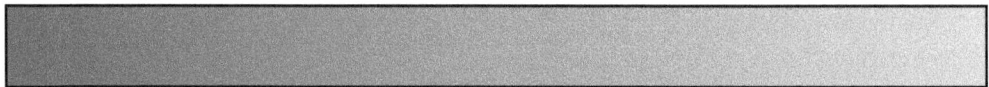

SAD   HAPPY

_____

_____

_____

_____

_____

IDEAS:

- play
- sleep
- social time
- quiet time
- spa/facial/massage etc.
- walk in nature
- daydreaming
- cook for myself
- order in

Self-Care Activity For Today

IDEAS:

- Taking care of myself gives me more to share with others.
- It is kind and wise to honor my limits.
- I allow myself to feel without judgment and release what no longer serves me.
- My thoughts can soften; I can choose peace in this moment.
- It is safe for me to slow down, breathe, and simply be.
- I give my body what it needs to feel nourished and supported.
- I listen with respect to the messages my body sends me.
- Rest is productive; my body heals and restores when I pause.

Today's Affirmation

TODAY'S DATE: _____

My goal(s) for today: I am grateful for...

_____   1. _____

_____   2. _____

_____   3. _____

_____   4. _____

_____   5. _____

How I feel today:
(mark with an X)

SAD   HAPPY

_____

_____

_____

_____

_____

_____

Self-Care Activity For Today

IDEAS:

➤ play
➤ sleep
➤ social time
➤ quiet time
➤ spa/facial/massage etc.
➤ walk in nature
➤ daydreaming
➤ cook for myself
➤ order in

Today's Affirmation

IDEAS:

➤ Taking care of myself gives me more to share with others.
➤ It is kind and wise to honor my limits.
➤ I allow myself to feel without judgment and release what no longer serves me.
➤ My thoughts can soften; I can choose peace in this moment.
➤ It is safe for me to slow down, breathe, and simply be.
➤ I give my body what it needs to feel nourished and supported.
➤ I listen with respect to the messages my body sends me.
➤ Rest is productive; my body heals and restores when I pause.

TODAY'S DATE: _____

My goal(s) for today: I am grateful for...

_____   1. _____

_____   2. _____

_____   3. _____

_____   4. _____

_____   5. _____

How I feel today:
(mark with an X)

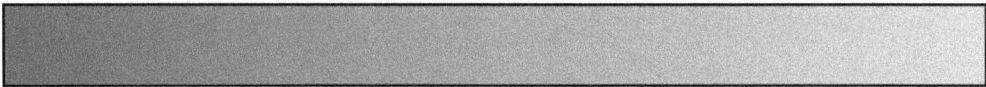

SAD   HAPPY

_____

_____

_____

_____

_____

IDEAS:

- play
- sleep
- social time
- quiet time
- spa/facial/massage etc.
- walk in nature
- daydreaming
- cook for myself
- order in

Self-Care Activity For Today

IDEAS:

- Taking care of myself gives me more to share with others.
- It is kind and wise to honor my limits.
- I allow myself to feel without judgment and release what no longer serves me.
- My thoughts can soften; I can choose peace in this moment.
- It is safe for me to slow down, breathe, and simply be.
- I give my body what it needs to feel nourished and supported.
- I listen with respect to the messages my body sends me.
- Rest is productive; my body heals and restores when I pause.

Today's Affirmation

TODAY'S DATE: _____

My goal(s) for today: I am grateful for...

_____   1. _____

_____   2. _____

_____   3. _____

_____   4. _____

_____   5. _____

How I feel today:
(mark with an X)

SAD   HAPPY

_____

_____

_____

_____

_____

IDEAS:

- play
- sleep
- social time
- quiet time
- spa/facial/massage etc.
- walk in nature
- daydreaming
- cook for myself
- order in

Self-Care Activity For Today

IDEAS:

- Taking care of myself gives me more to share with others.
- It is kind and wise to honor my limits.
- I allow myself to feel without judgment and release what no longer serves me.
- My thoughts can soften; I can choose peace in this moment.
- It is safe for me to slow down, breathe, and simply be.
- I give my body what it needs to feel nourished and supported.
- I listen with respect to the messages my body sends me.
- Rest is productive; my body heals and restores when I pause.

Today's Affirmation

TODAY'S DATE: _____

My goal(s) for today: I am grateful for...

_____   1. _____

_____   2. _____

_____   3. _____

_____   4. _____

_____   5. _____

How I feel today:
(mark with an X)

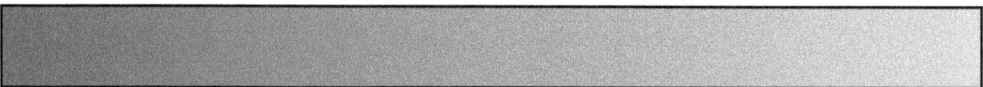

SAD   HAPPY

_____

_____

_____

_____

_____

IDEAS:

- play
- sleep
- social time
- quiet time
- spa/facial/massage etc.
- walk in nature
- daydreaming
- cook for myself
- order in

Self-Care Activity For Today

IDEAS:

- Taking care of myself gives me more to share with others.
- It is kind and wise to honor my limits.
- I allow myself to feel without judgment and release what no longer serves me.
- My thoughts can soften; I can choose peace in this moment.
- It is safe for me to slow down, breathe, and simply be.
- I give my body what it needs to feel nourished and supported.
- I listen with respect to the messages my body sends me.
- Rest is productive; my body heals and restores when I pause.

Today's Affirmation

TODAY'S DATE: _____

My goal(s) for today: I am grateful for...

_____   1. _____

_____   2. _____

_____   3. _____

_____   4. _____

_____   5. _____

How I feel today:
(mark with an X)

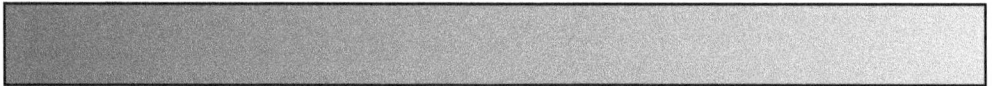

SAD   HAPPY

_____

_____

_____

_____

_____

IDEAS:

- play
- sleep
- social time
- quiet time
- spa/facial/massage etc.
- walk in nature
- daydreaming
- cook for myself
- order in

Self-Care Activity For Today

IDEAS:

- Taking care of myself gives me more to share with others.
- It is kind and wise to honor my limits.
- I allow myself to feel without judgment and release what no longer serves me.
- My thoughts can soften; I can choose peace in this moment.
- It is safe for me to slow down, breathe, and simply be.
- I give my body what it needs to feel nourished and supported.
- I listen with respect to the messages my body sends me.
- Rest is productive; my body heals and restores when I pause.

Today's Affirmation

TODAY'S DATE: _____

My goal(s) for today: I am grateful for...

_____   1. _____

_____   2. _____

_____   3. _____

_____   4. _____

_____   5. _____

How I feel today:
(mark with an X)

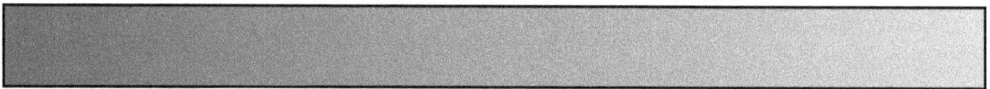

SAD   HAPPY

_____

_____

_____

_____

_____

_____

Self-Care Activity For Today

IDEAS:

- ➤ play
- ➤ sleep
- ➤ social time
- ➤ quiet time
- ➤ spa/facial/massage etc.
- ➤ walk in nature
- ➤ daydreaming
- ➤ cook for myself
- ➤ order in

Today's Affirmation

IDEAS:

- ➤ Taking care of myself gives me more to share with others.
- ➤ It is kind and wise to honor my limits.
- ➤ I allow myself to feel without judgment and release what no longer serves me.
- ➤ My thoughts can soften; I can choose peace in this moment.
- ➤ It is safe for me to slow down, breathe, and simply be.
- ➤ I give my body what it needs to feel nourished and supported.
- ➤ I listen with respect to the messages my body sends me.
- ➤ Rest is productive; my body heals and restores when I pause.

TODAY'S DATE: _____

My goal(s) for today: I am grateful for...

_____   1. _____

_____   2. _____

_____   3. _____

_____   4. _____

_____   5. _____

How I feel today:
(mark with an X)

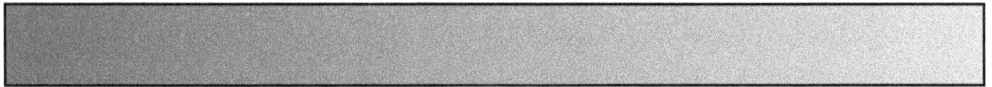

SAD   HAPPY

_____

_____

_____

_____

_____

IDEAS:

- ➤ play
- ➤ sleep
- ➤ social time
- ➤ quiet time
- ➤ spa/facial/massage etc.
- ➤ walk in nature
- ➤ daydreaming
- ➤ cook for myself
- ➤ order in

Self-Care Activity For Today

IDEAS:

- ➤ Taking care of myself gives me more to share with others.
- ➤ It is kind and wise to honor my limits.
- ➤ I allow myself to feel without judgment and release what no longer serves me.
- ➤ My thoughts can soften; I can choose peace in this moment.
- ➤ It is safe for me to slow down, breathe, and simply be.
- ➤ I give my body what it needs to feel nourished and supported.
- ➤ I listen with respect to the messages my body sends me.
- ➤ Rest is productive; my body heals and restores when I pause.

Today's Affirmation

TODAY'S DATE: _____

My goal(s) for today: I am grateful for...

_____   1. _____

_____   2. _____

_____   3. _____

_____   4. _____

_____   5. _____

How I feel today:
(mark with an X)

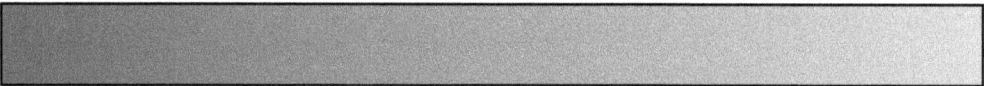

SAD   HAPPY

_____

_____

_____

_____

_____

IDEAS:

➤ play
➤ sleep
➤ social time
➤ quiet time
➤ spa/facial/massage etc.
➤ walk in nature
➤ daydreaming
➤ cook for myself
➤ order in

Self-Care Activity For Today

IDEAS:

➤ Taking care of myself gives me more to share with others.
➤ It is kind and wise to honor my limits.
➤ I allow myself to feel without judgment and release what no longer serves me.
➤ My thoughts can soften; I can choose peace in this moment.
➤ It is safe for me to slow down, breathe, and simply be.
➤ I give my body what it needs to feel nourished and supported.
➤ I listen with respect to the messages my body sends me.
➤ Rest is productive; my body heals and restores when I pause.

Today's Affirmation

TODAY'S DATE: _____

My goal(s) for today:

_____

_____

_____

_____

_____

I am grateful for...

1. _____

2. _____

3. _____

4. _____

5. _____

How I feel today:
(mark with an X)

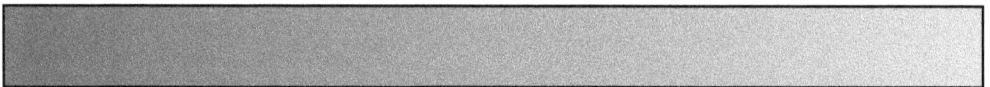

SAD   HAPPY

_____

_____

_____

_____

_____

IDEAS:

- play
- sleep
- social time
- quiet time
- spa/facial/massage etc.
- walk in nature
- daydreaming
- cook for myself
- order in

Self-Care Activity For Today

IDEAS:

- Taking care of myself gives me more to share with others.
- It is kind and wise to honor my limits.
- I allow myself to feel without judgment and release what no longer serves me.
- My thoughts can soften; I can choose peace in this moment.
- It is safe for me to slow down, breathe, and simply be.
- I give my body what it needs to feel nourished and supported.
- I listen with respect to the messages my body sends me.
- Rest is productive; my body heals and restores when I pause.

Today's Affirmation

My Everyday Pain Story

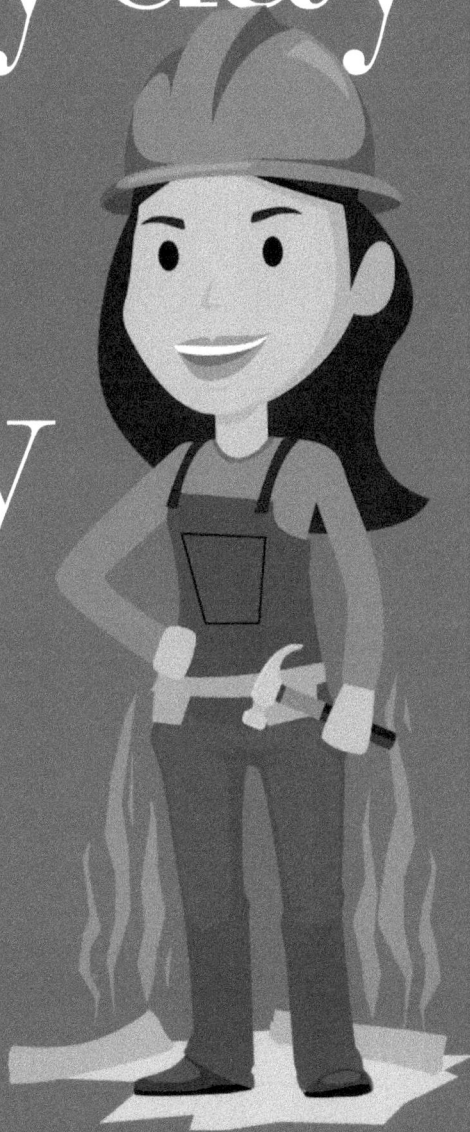

My Everyday Pain Story

When I release my pain, I feel...

_____

_____

_____

_____

_____

_____

_____

_____

_____

_____

_____

_____

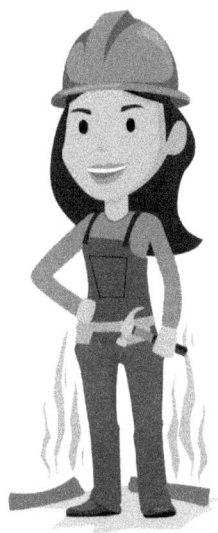

My Everyday Pain Story

When I have less pain, I look forward to...
doing/feeling/being:

_____

_____

_____

_____

_____

_____

_____

_____

_____

_____

_____

My Everyday Pain Story

When I have quieted my stress biology, I
look forward to...doing/feeling/being:

_____

_____

_____

_____

_____

_____

_____

_____

_____

_____

_____

_____

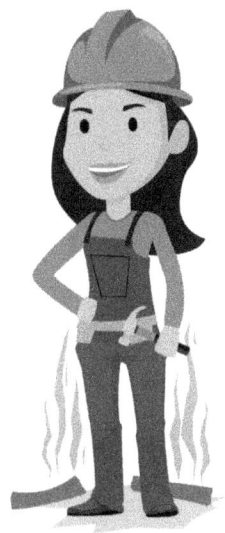

My Everyday Pain Story

When I am more grounded in my body, I look forward to...doing/feeling/being:

_____

_____

_____

_____

_____

_____

_____

_____

_____

_____

My Everyday Pain Story

My first or most memorable pain
experience or injury as a child

_____

_____

_____

_____

_____

_____

_____

_____

_____

_____

_____

_____

_____

_____

What part of me was hurt?

How did it happen?

Who was there with me or was I alone?

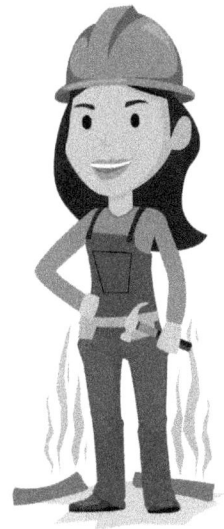

My Everyday Pain Story

If there was a parent, guardian, friend or teacher nearby, how did they react to my injury?

If I was alone at the time, how did I feel about that?

Were any of these feelings present: shame, blame, anger, fear, embarrassment, humor, achievement?

Notes:

_____

_____

_____

_____

_____

_____

_____

_____

_____

_____

_____

_____

_____

My Everyday Pain Story

Notes:

_____

_____

_____

_____

_____

_____

_____

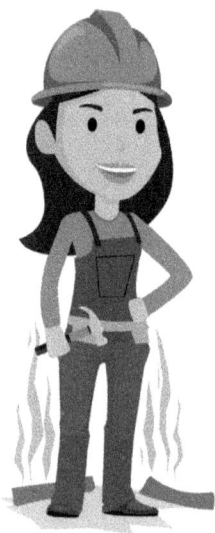

_____

_____

_____

_____

_____

My Monthly Check In

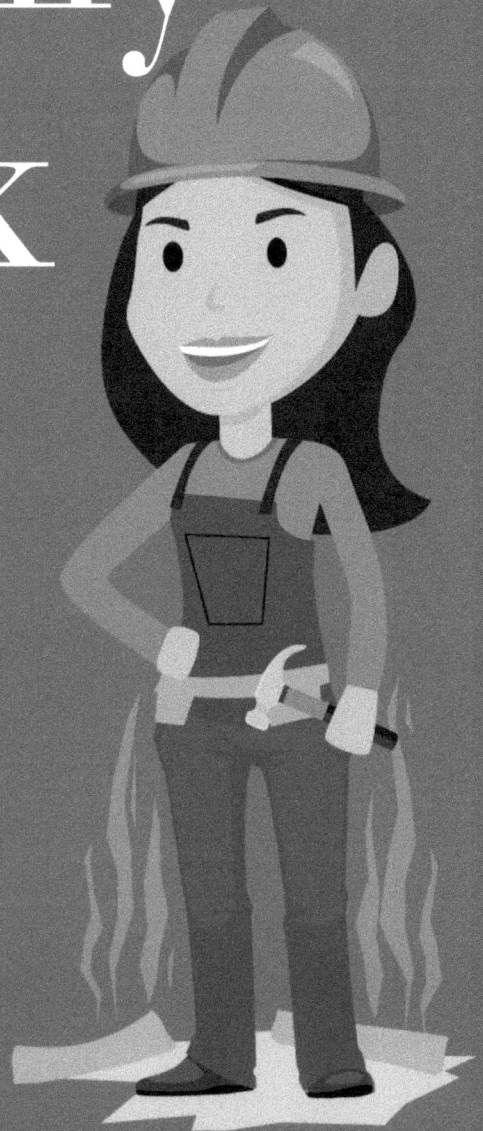

THE CHECK IN

How are you feeling?

TODAY'S DATE: _____

PAIN LOCATION:
(circle one)

Neck   Neck/Shoulder   Shoulder/Upper Back   Mid Back/Torso/Ribs

Low Back   Low Back/Hip   Hip/Buttock/Thigh

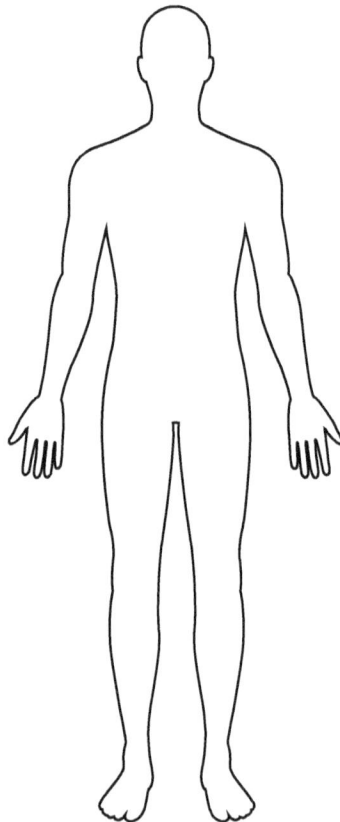

Use this figure to color or shade-in the area of your pain however you like.

HOW MUCH PAIN TODAY?

Circle the face below that best expresses your discomfort:

Wong-Baker FACES® Pain Rating Scale

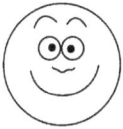 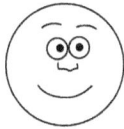 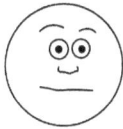 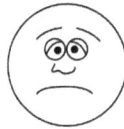 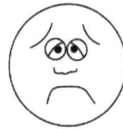 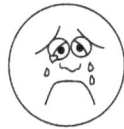

0	**2**	**4**	**6**	**8**	**10**
No Pain	A Little Pain	A Little More Pain	Even More Pain	A Whole Lot Of Pain	Worst Pain

Notes:

_____

_____

_____

_____

_____

_____

_____

_____

THE CHECK IN

How are you feeling?

TODAY'S DATE: _____

PAIN LOCATION:
(circle one)

Neck   Neck/Shoulder   Shoulder/Upper Back   Mid Back/Torso/Ribs

Low Back   Low Back/Hip   Hip/Buttock/Thigh

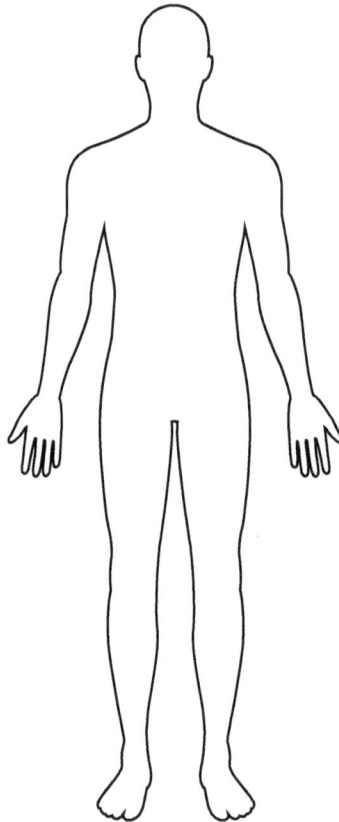

Use this figure to color or shade-in the area of your pain however you like.

HOW MUCH PAIN TODAY?

Circle the face below that best expresses your discomfort:

Wong-Baker FACES® Pain Rating Scale

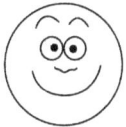 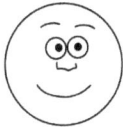 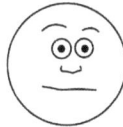 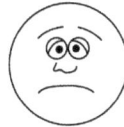 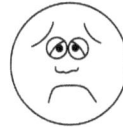 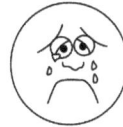

0	2	4	6	8	10
No Pain	A Little Pain	A Little More Pain	Even More Pain	A Whole Lot Of Pain	Worst Pain

Notes:

_____

_____

_____

_____

_____

_____

_____

_____

THE CHECK IN

How are you feeling?

TODAY'S DATE: _____

PAIN LOCATION:
(circle one)

Neck   Neck/Shoulder   Shoulder/Upper Back   Mid Back/Torso/Ribs

Low Back   Low Back/Hip   Hip/Buttock/Thigh

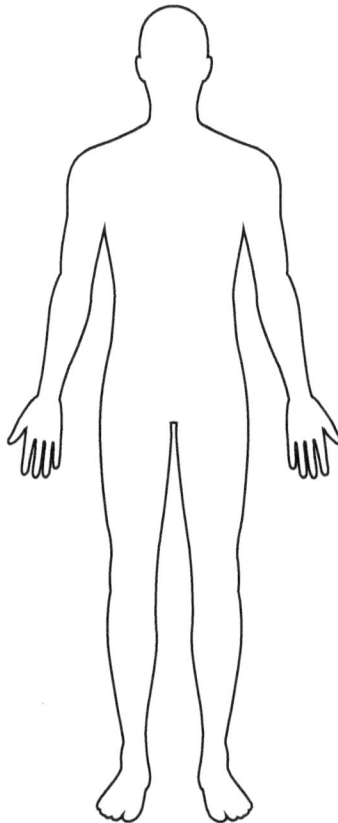

Use this figure to color or shade-in the area of your pain however you like.

HOW MUCH PAIN TODAY?

Circle the face below that best expresses your discomfort:

Wong-Baker FACES® Pain Rating Scale

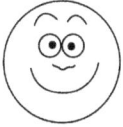 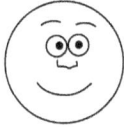 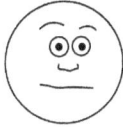 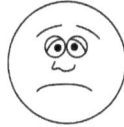 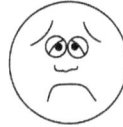 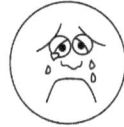

0	2	4	6	8	10
No Pain	A Little Pain	A Little More Pain	Even More Pain	A Whole Lot Of Pain	Worst Pain

Notes:

_____

_____

_____

_____

_____

_____

_____

_____

THE CHECK IN

How are you feeling?

TODAY'S DATE: _____

PAIN LOCATION:
(circle one)

Neck   Neck/Shoulder   Shoulder/Upper Back   Mid Back/Torso/Ribs

Low Back   Low Back/Hip   Hip/Buttock/Thigh

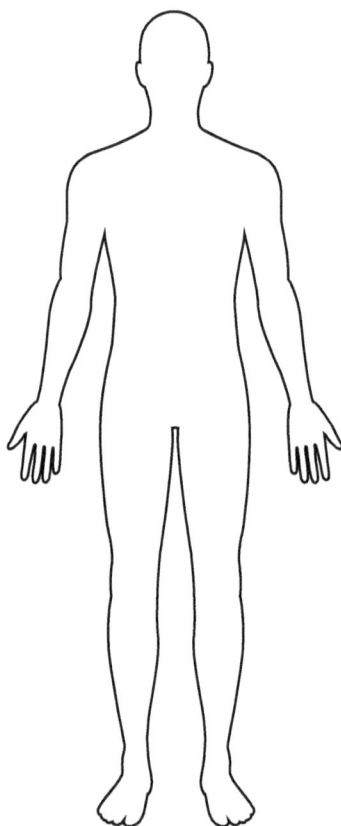

Use this figure to color or shade-in the area of your pain however you like.

HOW MUCH PAIN TODAY?

Circle the face below that best expresses your discomfort:

Wong-Baker FACES® Pain Rating Scale

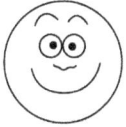 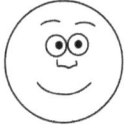 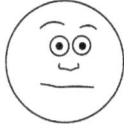 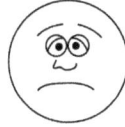 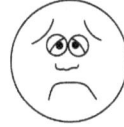 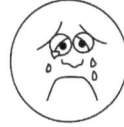

0	**2**	**4**	**6**	**8**	**10**
No Pain	A Little Pain	A Little More Pain	Even More Pain	A Whole Lot Of Pain	Worst Pain

Notes:

_____

_____

_____

_____

_____

_____

_____

_____

How are you feeling?

TODAY'S DATE: _____

PAIN LOCATION:
(circle one)

Neck   Neck/Shoulder   Shoulder/Upper Back   Mid Back/Torso/Ribs

Low Back   Low Back/Hip   Hip/Buttock/Thigh

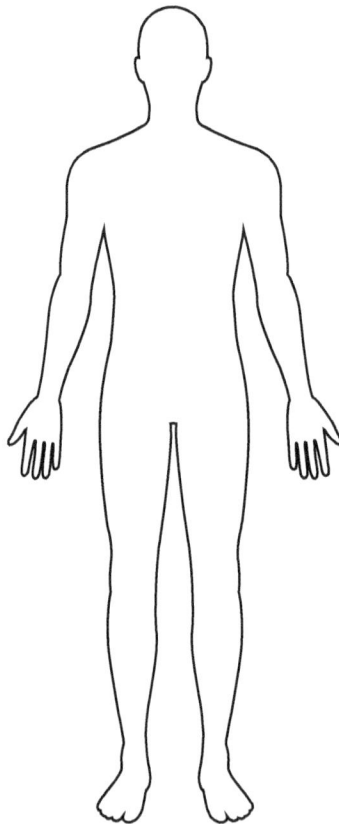

Use this figure to color or shade-in the area of your pain however you like.

HOW MUCH PAIN TODAY?

Circle the face below that best expresses your discomfort:

Wong-Baker FACES® Pain Rating Scale

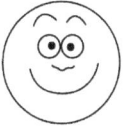 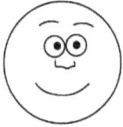 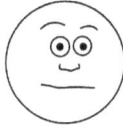 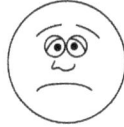 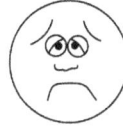 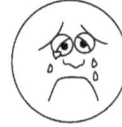

0	2	4	6	8	10
No Pain	A Little Pain	A Little More Pain	Even More Pain	A Whole Lot Of Pain	Worst Pain

Notes:

_____

_____

_____

_____

_____

_____

_____

_____

THE CHECK IN

How are you feeling?

TODAY'S DATE: _____

PAIN LOCATION:
(circle one)

Neck   Neck/Shoulder   Shoulder/Upper Back   Mid Back/Torso/Ribs

Low Back   Low Back/Hip   Hip/Buttock/Thigh

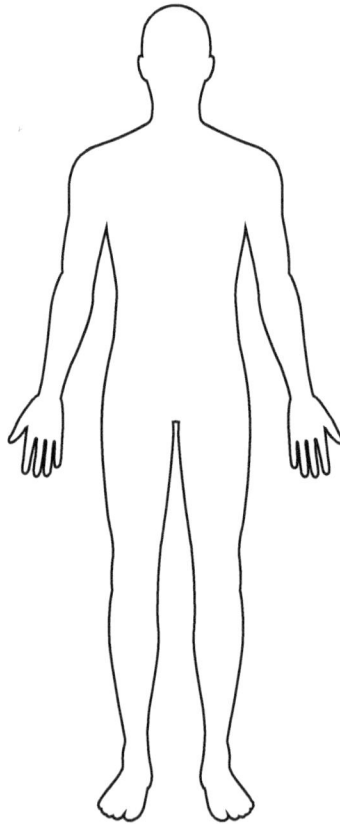

Use this figure to color or shade-in the area of your pain however you like.

HOW MUCH PAIN TODAY?

Circle the face below that best expresses your discomfort:

Wong-Baker FACES® Pain Rating Scale

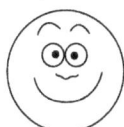 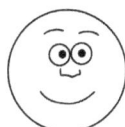 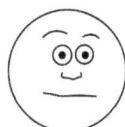 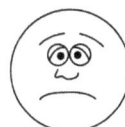 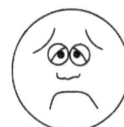 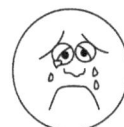

0	**2**	**4**	**6**	**8**	**10**
No Pain	A Little Pain	A Little More Pain	Even More Pain	A Whole Lot Of Pain	Worst Pain

Notes:

_____

_____

_____

_____

_____

_____

_____

_____

THE CHECK IN

How are you feeling?

TODAY'S DATE: _____

PAIN LOCATION:
(circle one)

Neck   Neck/Shoulder   Shoulder/Upper Back   Mid Back/Torso/Ribs

Low Back   Low Back/Hip   Hip/Buttock/Thigh

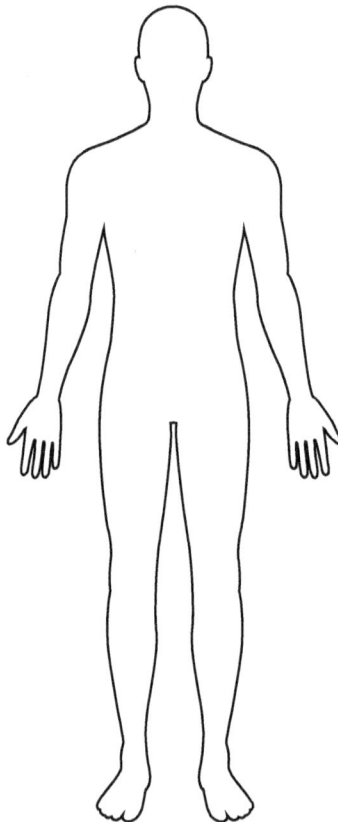

Use this figure to color or shade-in the area of your pain however you like.

HOW MUCH PAIN TODAY?

Circle the face below that best expresses your discomfort:

Wong-Baker FACES® Pain Rating Scale

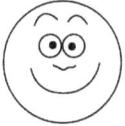 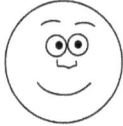 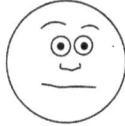 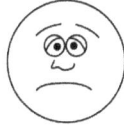 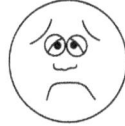 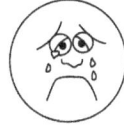

0	2	4	6	8	10
No Pain	A Little Pain	A Little More Pain	Even More Pain	A Whole Lot Of Pain	Worst Pain

Notes:

_____

_____

_____

_____

_____

_____

_____

_____

THE CHECK IN

How are you feeling?

TODAY'S DATE: _____

PAIN LOCATION:
(circle one)

Neck   Neck/Shoulder   Shoulder/Upper Back   Mid Back/Torso/Ribs

Low Back   Low Back/Hip   Hip/Buttock/Thigh

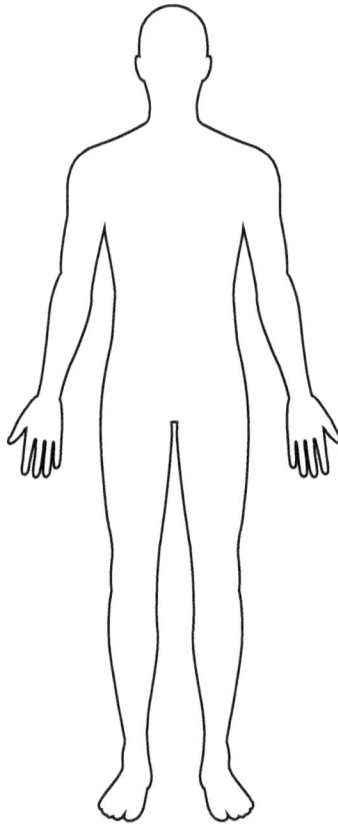

Use this figure to color or shade-in the area of your pain however you like.

HOW MUCH PAIN TODAY?

Circle the face below that best expresses your discomfort:

Wong-Baker FACES® Pain Rating Scale

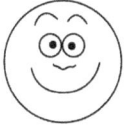 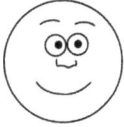 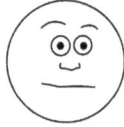 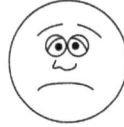 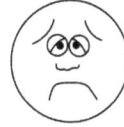 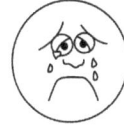

0	**2**	**4**	**6**	**8**	**10**
No Pain	A Little Pain	A Little More Pain	Even More Pain	A Whole Lot Of Pain	Worst Pain

Notes:

_____

_____

_____

_____

_____

_____

_____

_____

THE CHECK IN

How are you feeling?

TODAY'S DATE: _____

PAIN LOCATION:
(circle one)

Neck   Neck/Shoulder   Shoulder/Upper Back   Mid Back/Torso/Ribs

Low Back   Low Back/Hip   Hip/Buttock/Thigh

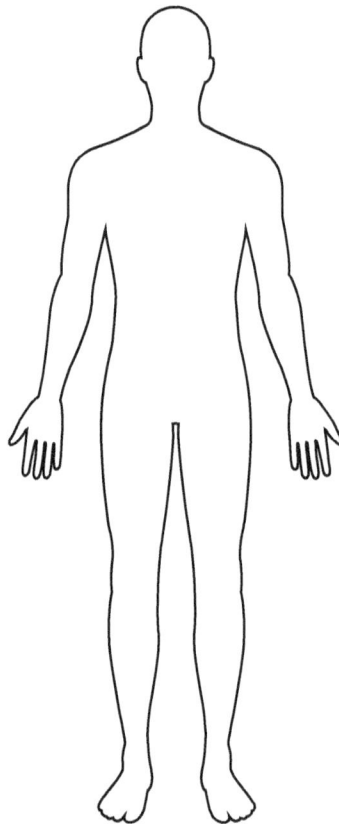

Use this figure to color or shade-in the area of your pain however you like.

HOW MUCH PAIN TODAY?

Circle the face below that best expresses your discomfort:

Wong-Baker FACES® Pain Rating Scale

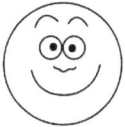 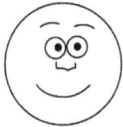 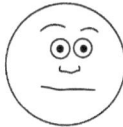 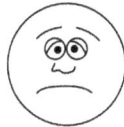 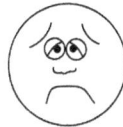 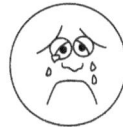

0	2	4	6	8	10
No Pain	A Little Pain	A Little More Pain	Even More Pain	A Whole Lot Of Pain	Worst Pain

Notes:

_____

_____

_____

_____

_____

_____

_____

_____

THE CHECK IN

How are you feeling?

TODAY'S DATE: _____

PAIN LOCATION:
(circle one)

Neck   Neck/Shoulder   Shoulder/Upper Back   Mid Back/Torso/Ribs

Low Back   Low Back/Hip   Hip/Buttock/Thigh

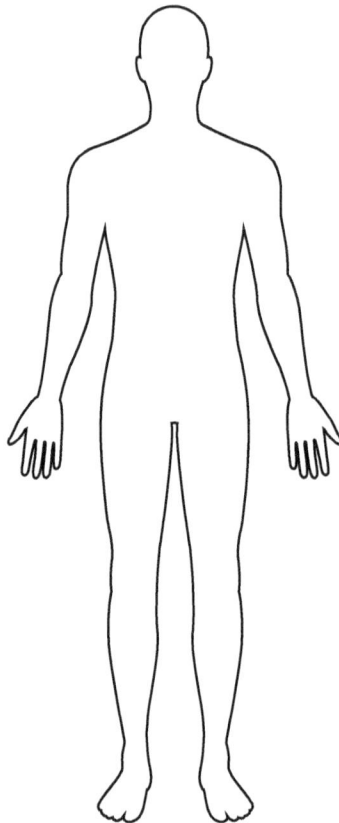

Use this figure to color or shade-in the area of your pain however you like.

HOW MUCH PAIN TODAY?

Circle the face below that best expresses your discomfort:

Wong-Baker FACES® Pain Rating Scale

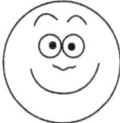 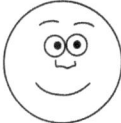 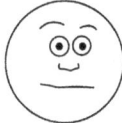 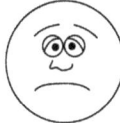 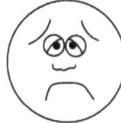 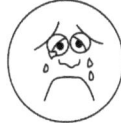

0	2	4	6	8	10
No Pain	A Little Pain	A Little More Pain	Even More Pain	A Whole Lot Of Pain	Worst Pain

Notes:

_____

_____

_____

_____

_____

_____

_____

_____

THE CHECK IN

How are you feeling?

TODAY'S DATE: _____

PAIN LOCATION:
(circle one)

Neck   Neck/Shoulder   Shoulder/Upper Back   Mid Back/Torso/Ribs

Low Back   Low Back/Hip   Hip/Buttock/Thigh

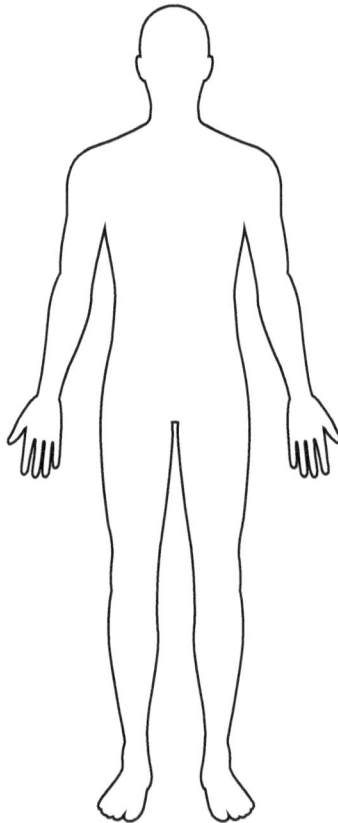

Use this figure to color or shade-in the area of your pain however you like.

HOW MUCH PAIN TODAY?

Circle the face below that best expresses your discomfort:

Wong-Baker FACES® Pain Rating Scale

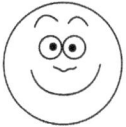 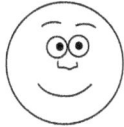 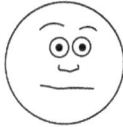 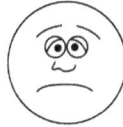 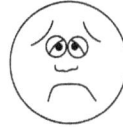 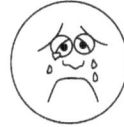

0	**2**	**4**	**6**	**8**	**10**
No Pain	A Little Pain	A Little More Pain	Even More Pain	A Whole Lot Of Pain	Worst Pain

Notes:

_____

_____

_____

_____

_____

_____

_____

_____

THE CHECK IN

How are you feeling?

TODAY'S DATE: _____

PAIN LOCATION:
(circle one)

Neck   Neck/Shoulder   Shoulder/Upper Back   Mid Back/Torso/Ribs

Low Back   Low Back/Hip   Hip/Buttock/Thigh

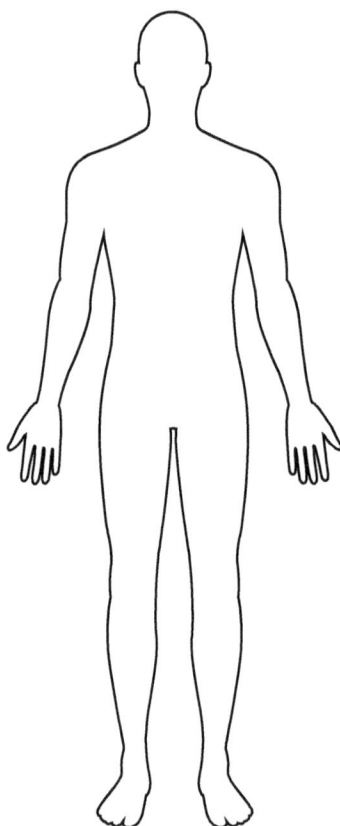

Use this figure to color or shade-in the area of your pain however you like.

HOW MUCH PAIN TODAY?

Circle the face below that best expresses your discomfort:

Wong-Baker FACES® Pain Rating Scale

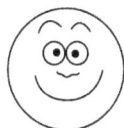 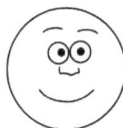 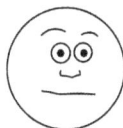 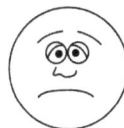 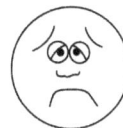 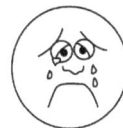

0	2	4	6	8	10
No Pain	A Little Pain	A Little More Pain	Even More Pain	A Whole Lot Of Pain	Worst Pain

Notes:

_____

_____

_____

_____

_____

_____

_____

_____

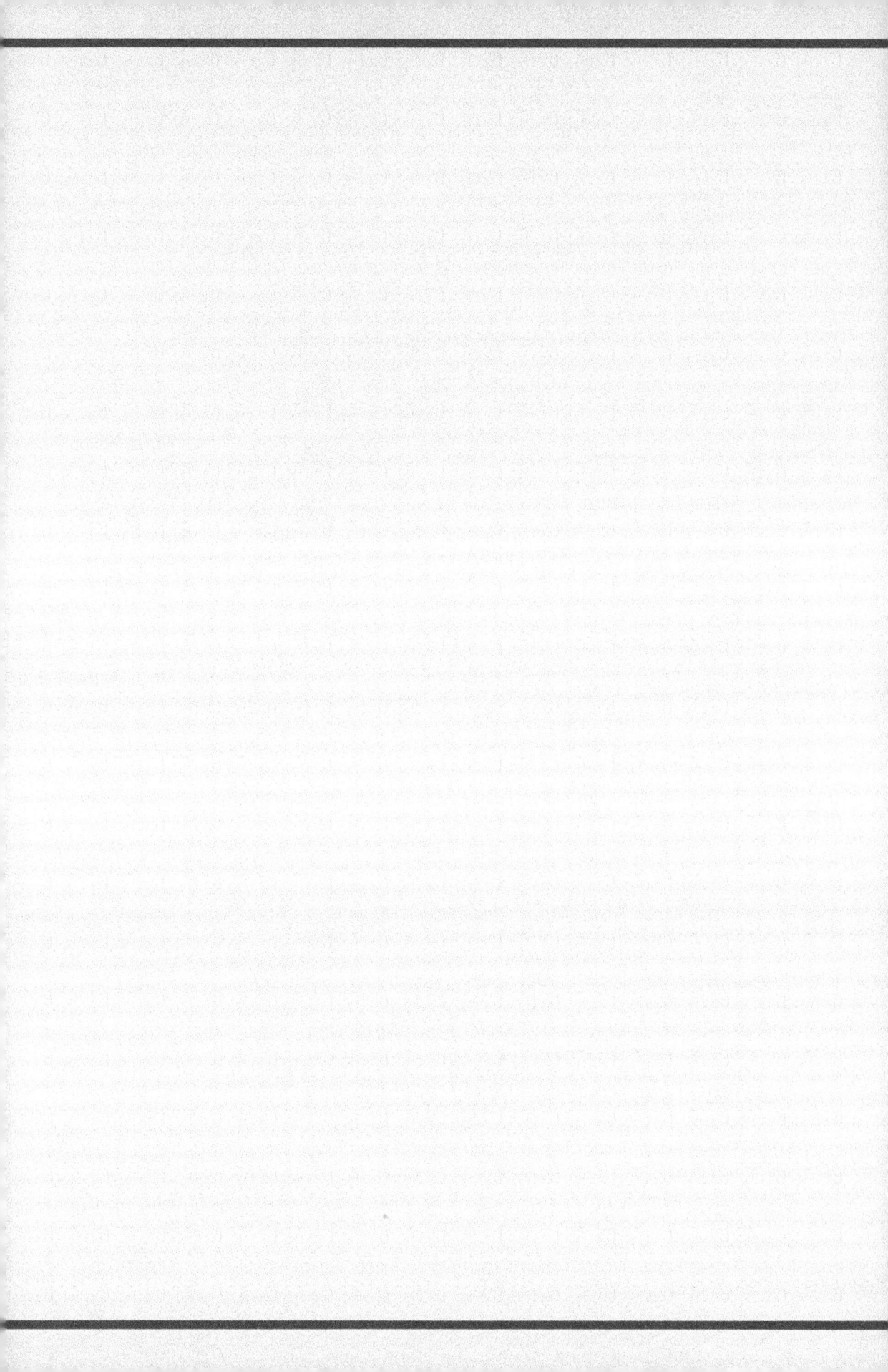

What the Pros Say

A Question and Answer
Session with the Pros

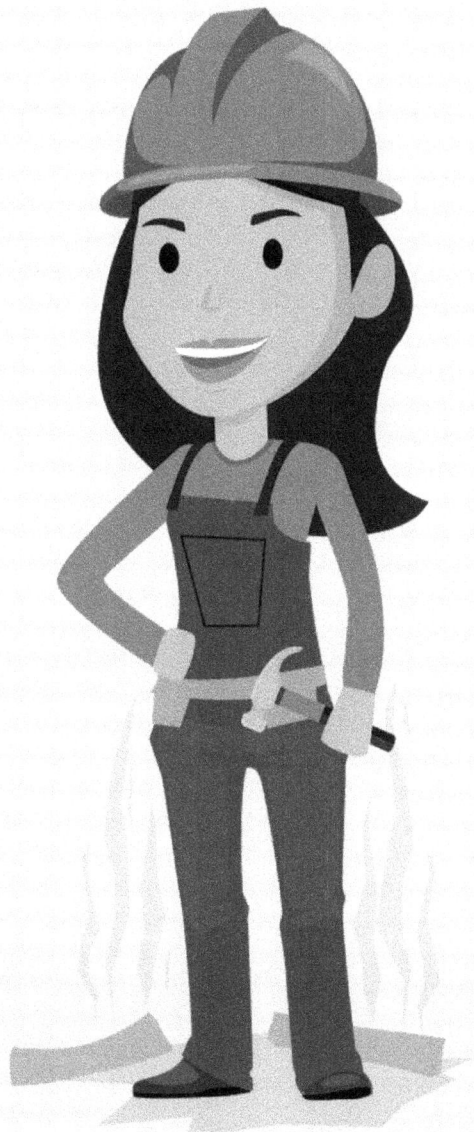

WHAT THE PROS SAY

WHAT FOLLOWS NEXT IS A COLLECTION of perspectives from a small sampling of providers with experience in behavioral health. These five voices are practitioners local to Seattle, Washington, who kindly responded to my request for contributions to this book series. I'm sharing their insights about treating pain specifically from a psychosocial point of view. I urge you to use some of the questions addressed here as a jumping-off point as you consider your next phase in the pain repair process, which may include exploring your unique social, emotional and psychological needs.

Please note that none of this is an endorsement for or against a specific modality or method. Rather, this section will primarily show you a small sampling of existing care options. At the end of this chapter, you'll see my personal take on what the bottom line might be. While each interview was unique, there are a few common threads that you might also detect as you read through them.

MEET THE PROS

Barbara Rose Chateaubriand, MA

barbararosechateaubriand.com

Barbara Rose Chateaubriand, M.A. has been a psychotherapist in private practice since1991. She is a certified in EMDR (Eye Movement Desensitization and Reprocessing therapy). She has been working with clients with trauma most of that time and finds that the mind/body connection is profound.

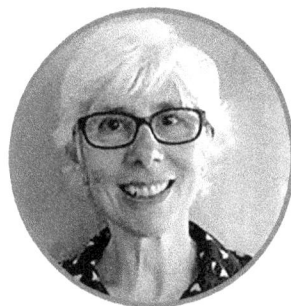

Alex Alexander ND LMHC

painalternativesclinic.com

Alex Alexander, ND LMHC is a specialist in osteopathic manipulative techniques and structural balancing for acute and chronic painful conditions and offers psychotherapy and medication support for chronic pain, traumatic stress, depression and anxiety, grief, and trauma recovery.

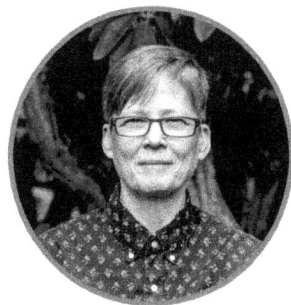

Meet the Pros

Mark Grant MA

overcomingpain.com

Mark Grant MA is an Australian psychologist/researcher. Mark has 30 years experience as a clinician. Mark is particularly interested in the impact of stress on health and the involvement of the brain in stress. Reflecting his origins as the son of an artist and an engineer, he likes to take a creative but practical approach to creating tools for undoing the effects of severe stress; i.e., strategies that harness innate brain capabilities. He is definitely someone who is prepared to look outside traditionally accepted ways of thinking and doings things in his profession. He is motivated to do what works best for his clients rather than what is in some text-book. In addition to various research papers, apps and other audio downloads he is the author of 'Change Your Brain Change Your Pain' (self-help() and 'Pain Control with EMDR' (clinical treatment manual).

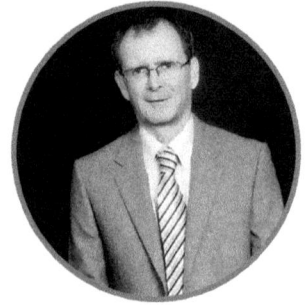

Tracy Rekart

tracyrekart.com

Tracy Rekart has a BA in Art History and Women Studies, an MS in Applied Behavioral Science, is a Master Somatic Coach, is deeply steeped in Eastern modalities, climbs rocks and mountains, and has been meditating and practicing yoga for over 25 years.

Tracy infuses soul-based questions, with actionable skill-based tools, and somatic bodywork and movement practices to support you to navigate the path through the unknown and toward your unique ecological niche (Bill Plotkin).

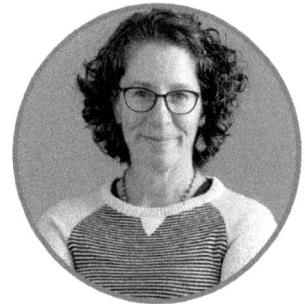

Ilene Dillon MSW

emotionalmasteryforlife.com

Ilene Dillon, MSW is the founder of Emotional Mastery for Life. She is dedicated to helping the world get Emotions in Motion, leading people to Mastery over Emotions. A 45-year Marriage and Family Therapist in California, Professional Speaker, Author, and former host of "Full Power Living," Ilene is currently writing a series of books, "Emotions in Motion."

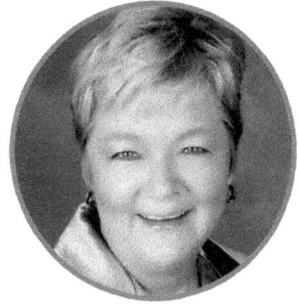

ASK THE PROS

Ask the Pros

How would you describe your role to someone seeking help for chronic recurring aches and pains?

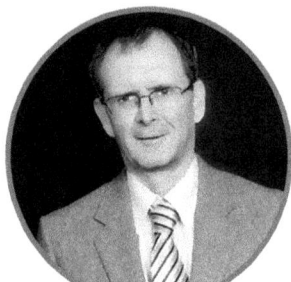

Mark Grant, MA

To assist pain sufferer to feel less overwhelmed by the pain. To address any trauma or personality issues that might be undermining their ability to cope. To help sufferer understand pain as a problem that can be managed. To help sufferer discover resources within themselves to combat pain. To understand meaning of pain both somatically and existentially. To develop a more integrated sense of self where pain is part of but not dominant feature.

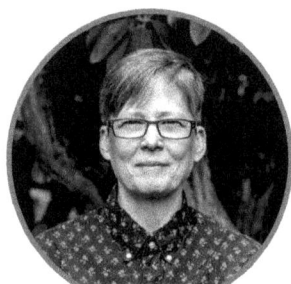

Alex Alexander, ND LMHC

I am first and foremost a partner in your wellness. I believe in you, and I believe that you can and will feel better. I have been fortunate to receive the education and experience to grasp what may be going on with you neurologically, anatomically and physiologically; and I honor and accept that you've been given hope before that things could improve and not actually seen that improvement happen. I acknowledge that you are the expert in you and that I am the expert in listening and applying the treatments or modalities that I believe are right for your individual situation. I strive to help you find a program that will give you a chance to manage your pain so you can enjoy your life. Pain is never one thing; and as such, one thing alone won't likely make it manageable. Chronic pain care is a process, and you are not alone. I have expectations, you have expectations, and together we will manage our expectations and even challenge our current thoughts about what's possible in order to help you move closer to the version of yourself you've been missing.

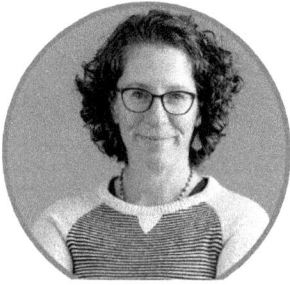

Tracy Rekart

I Facilitate the processing of historical shaping that often leads to aches and pains. I do this through goal centered conversation, listening for the person underneath he words. I help people learn to move more with ease through teaching movement practices that reveal us to ourselves and beg the question: is this who I want to be? How I want to move through the world? And I work to help people notice the holding patterns that live in the body through bodywork, releasing the held patterns which allow people to feel themselves unrestricted. In conjunction with conversation and movement, this creates a full picture of where a person wants to go, what physically and physiologically prevents them from going there, and then lets them feel the body that would get them there. Through this experience, people feel where they want to be/go, and then we create practices and structures that help them get there.

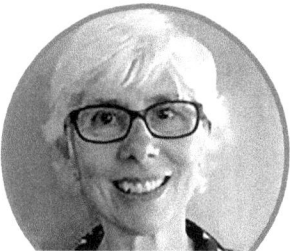

Barbara Rose
Chateaubriand, MA

Generally, if someone is referred to me with chronic aches and pains, the referring caregiver has a concern that the pain might be related to psychological issues. My job is to help the client untangle that, and to work on understanding and healing the psychological aspects.

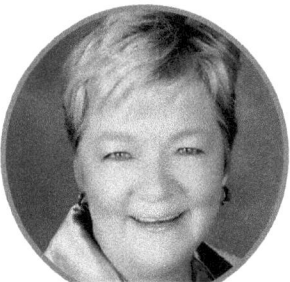

Ilene Dillon, MSW

I'm a Clinical Social Worker. My inquiry would be regarding the emotional component of such pain, as well as referral to pain-treating agencies, doctors or other health centers.

Ask the Pros

How do you feel about working with patients who are concurrently also receiving other care (acupuncture, massage, chiropractic, physical therapy, psychotherapy, other)? Do you find it affects outcomes positively or negatively?

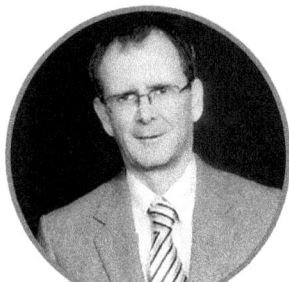

Mark Grant, MA

I feel pleased to work with patients who are receiving other care because chronic pain is a mind-body-spirit problem, which requires a multi-dimensional approach. I find that most adjunctive treatments have a positive overall impact if applied correctly and with sympathy to patients' abilities and needs. I advocate an integrative approach because I feel that disintegration (whether individually or systemically) is often at the core of chronic pain conditions.

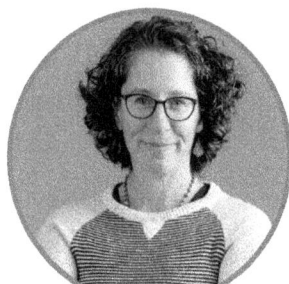

Tracy Rekart

I strongly believe that people must find a variety of practitioners to support their growth and health. I think working on many fronts to return to healing is important. I also think that taking time in between these practitioner visits to digest, either through the body or both body and mind, the work that was done is important before getting more work. If we do not take time to digest, we can often add more confusion to the system. I believe experienced practitioners can sense this and work to adjust their treatment or suggest digestion time. Mostly, I think the person has to have a clear idea of what problem they are trying to solve or what question they are trying to answer. Then the person must be ready to take what they learn and lightly experiment with it to see if or how it fits into their goals and needs. If people are shooting at the side of a barn by going from practitioner to practitioner, without knowing specifically why, or at least generally why, and trying to decipher this, I think it can do harm in further confusing or even injuring the person.

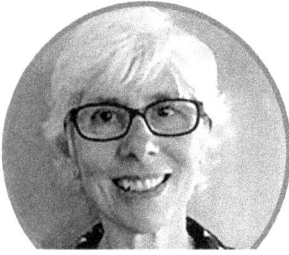

Barbara Rose
Chateaubriand, MA

I am always glad when my clients are working on solving their problems and regaining health and equilibrium in multiple ways. I find that when my client is truly motivated to move forward in their healing, the most positive outcomes occur. Many people cannot afford to be in multiple therapies at one time, and then I encourage them to figure out what is most acute at the time and work on that.

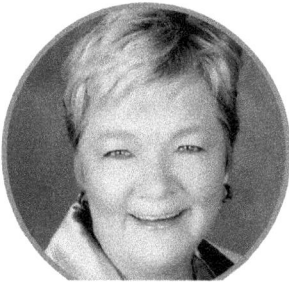

Ilene Dillon, MSW

Positively. I think it's a great thing, and not done frequently enough. We need to work as teams. No one person/practitioner can have all the answers.

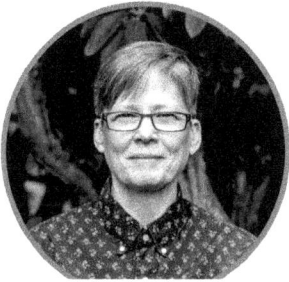

Alex Alexander, ND LMHC

Fine. It takes a village. Really. There is no place for ego (or egocentrism about a profession) when helping people become better versions of themselves. We are all valid.

Ask the Pros

Do you counsel patients/clients about how to coordinate integrative care with other professionals? If so, what are your common recommendations?

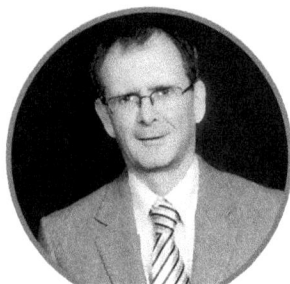

I recommend to patients that they consider other treatment modalities (physio, chiro, massage, etc.). For many patients, it is a new thing to have to take such a proactive interest in their own well-being. For patients with a history of trauma or abuse, it may be a difficult thing to accept or believe, and they may need trauma therapy such as EMDR to resolve any emotional blockages or beliefs (e.g., shame, 'I am not worth it') to doing this.

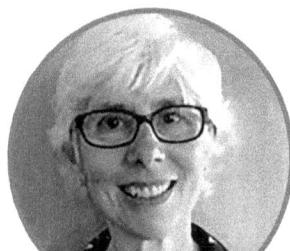

Mark Grant, MA

If I believe it might be helpful to a client to have their caregivers communicate, I talk with them about it, and if they are open, encourage them to sign a mutual release of confidentiality, and to let their other caregivers know.

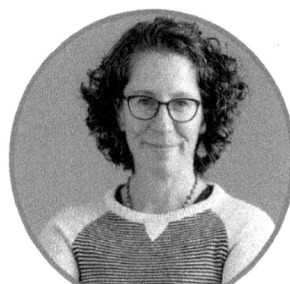

Barbara Rose Chateaubriand, MA

If people are seeking multiple opinions, I often help them get clear on their desired goal to see which practitioners may be the best fit for the moment. The ones that will help them answer, define, and get clarity on the question they are asking. I also ask them which practitioner listens or speaks to the part of them that is most in need of support right now. They often know this and can answer the question. Then I ask them the degree of processing they can or are willing to do. And go from there to illustrate through their telling of their own story, the best line of action for them.

Tracy Rekart

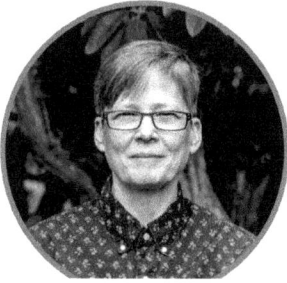

Alex Alexander, ND LMHC

Yes. I recommend acupuncture, counseling, craniosacral, and spiritual practices if the patient mentions they are so inclined, chiropractic medicine, and psychiatry when needed. I also send people to naturopaths, osteopaths, allopaths, and other specialists, if indicated.

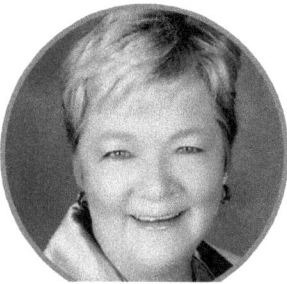

Ilene Dillon, MSW

Not really.

Ask the Pros

Do you make lifestyle recommendations? If so, are there one or two that you recommend more often than others and why?

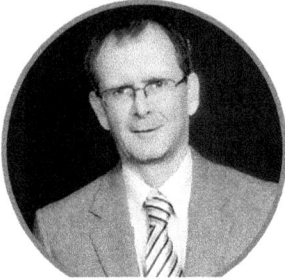

Mark Grant, MA

Yes.

Exercise – apart from its physical benefits, exercise is known to facilitate positive emotions and enhance neuroplasticity.

Goals – individual personal goals give life purpose and meaning, and reduce the amount of space occupied by the pain.

Supportive relationships – Having supportive relationships provides a buffer against the distress of pain.

Hobbies/enjoyable activities – Enjoyable activities stimulate positive emotions, distract a person from pain.

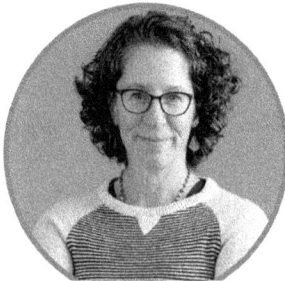

Tracy Rekart

Yes. Meditation. Paying attention to your breathing. That is my go-to. Or some sort of mindfulness practice. In order to heal, we must get to know the self. Until then, we are just putting Band-Aids on the end of a faucet that is turned on. If people do not know where they begin and end, it is hard to feel if any treatment/process is working. I also ask them who their support team is. This is an often-neglected part of healing. If they do not have one, then the healing work they do may not take hold or be able to be sustained. And noticing this and speaking it out loud is often startling, and the first step to making a change in partnership, friendship, or our family system, and drinking water. I often recommend that they drink lots of water to process our sessions. More than they normally drink, and then ask that they continue this practice to flush things out of their system.

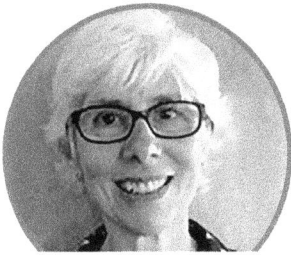

Barbara Rose
Chateaubriand, MA

If I believe it might be helpful, I will make suggestions regarding lifestyle. The most common are exercise, diet, vitamin D, and safe human interaction.

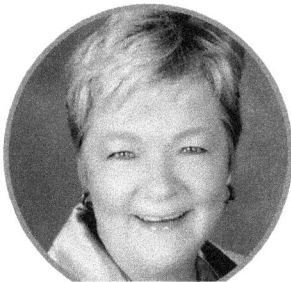

Ilene Dillon, MSW

I tend to consider food and nutritional alternatives, seek out nutritionists for referral, and refer to alternative herbs and supplements I know have been helpful to others.

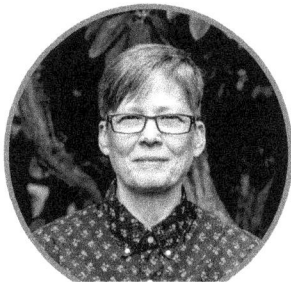

Alex Alexander, ND LMHC

The short answer is yes. There are some concerns in how this is delivered, in my opinion, because I never want my patients to feel unsupported or judged. I may gently suggest something that has some bang for the buck, so the patient is compelled to perhaps consider other suggestions they have heard, but I try and get them to tell me what they already know they need, which is more often the case. The CBT for chronic pain program I use has lifestyle mod built in, so slow and steady exercise, sleep hygiene, non-toxic relationships, anti-inflammatory eating habits, more water, smoking cessation, moderate to minimal EtOH is all built in. Those are the important ones for me.

Ask the Pros

Are there any other common "homework" tasks (behavior modification) that you require of your patients/clients while under your care?

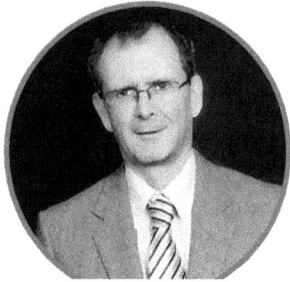
Mark Grant, MA

I rarely give patients homework. I give them resources (e.g., audio downloads, pain control exercises) which I usually demonstrate in session - if the patient has found the exercise helpful in session, they will do it without need for homework. For example, I demonstrate the use of audio bilateral stimulation (a treatment element of EMDR) to assuage anxiety and pain in session. If the patient experiences some relief, I give them details of one of my apps (Anxiety Release or Sleep Restore) with the suggestion to practice this at home. In my view, if you have to give the patient homework, it's putting the horse before the cart If you create a positive, resourced state in the patient, they will do what they need to do without homework

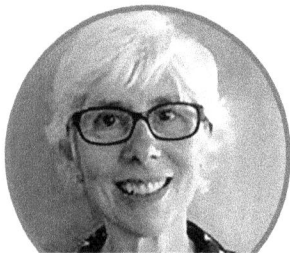
Barbara Rose
Chateaubriand, MA

While I do give homework to my clients, there are not any that are specially required. It is on a case-by-case basis.

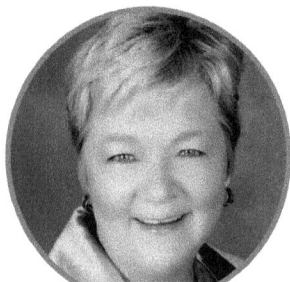
Ilene Dillon, MSW

Yes, making careful observation of what happens with their problem, and how they respond to it. Looking for habits that may need changing.

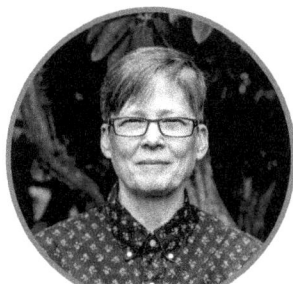

Alex Alexander, ND LMHC

If they are in the CBT-CP program with me, then yes. If not, I gauge the patient's willingness and readiness first before homework comes out. I use a lot of therapy tools that are free and easy to download, and TED talks, YouTube, books, etc. If it's a pure homework assignment I need to give, I try and make it all about the patient so they feel more deeply heard and supported by having another chance to talk about themselves and their experiences. Homework is a tough one, I think, because some patients expect it and others will never ever do it and feel harmed by their perceived failure. Setting expectations is key for my patients if I think I am going to need them to do homework. I have to get their buy-in first.

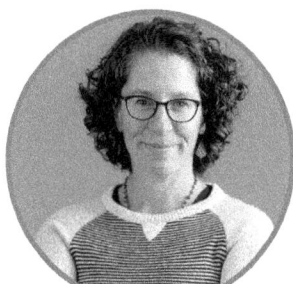

Tracy Rekart

Common homework is meditation or a centering practice. Something that helps people get to know themselves. The person underneath the role or veneer that we often call the self. Usually, there is a goal that the person is trying to achieve. Wanting to be pain-free, wanting a new role or direction, or wanting to be a more settled person. Being able to know themselves as centered and what the circumstances are around feeling centered. How they become centered. What helps them feel that way. How they get out or what triggers them out of that place. This helps people see a connection between their flow state and their maybe pain state.

Ask the Pros

Has there ever been a situation where you would turn someone away or re-direct them to a different therapy/modality? If so, please explain the circumstances.

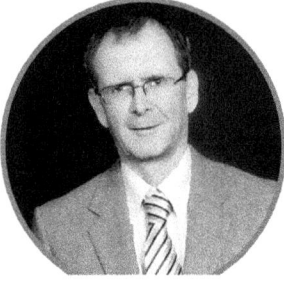

If a person's pain and suffering are severe and have not responded to my input, I have occasionally referred them to a pain specialist to review medication options. If a person needs a homework -based approach I refer them to pain specialists who use CBT (not often) If a person's pain is not responding significantly to my input I regularly refer them to other therapeutic modalities I believe that some people who might not respond to psychological interventions are more likely to respond to non-cognitive approaches such as massage or exercise.

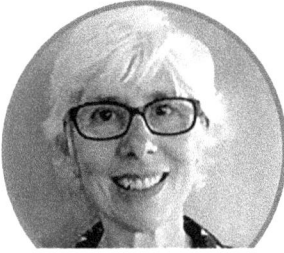

Mark Grant, MA

Yes, if I am not qualified to help them, or if it is not a good match to work together.

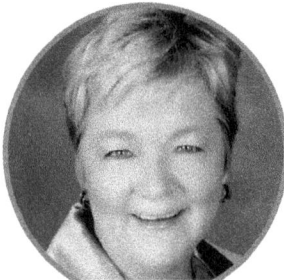

Barbara Rose
Chateaubriand, MA

Yes. There are some issues better treated by others. I have frequently referred people for alcohol and substance abuse, for psychosis, in particular.

Ilene Dillon, MSW

I am not a huge fan of therapeutic injections that involve taking out blood and reinjecting the spun cells, so that is probably the biggest one I dissuade patients from using, but never in a harsh or judgey way. It's more like "well, I get why that would be appealing because it's your own cells, etc., and I really want it to be a miracle cure also; however, I am waiting for a little more science and research since I don't know enough about it to recommend it." I can't really ever feel good about bashing another professional's work, even if I think it's terrifying. I also don't want my patients in danger, though, so if it's super sketchy and the patient asks me for my opinion, I will give it with a disclaimer such as "no, I wouldn't do that personally because I don't know enough about it, so perhaps you could consult with someone who knows more than I about this particular modality."

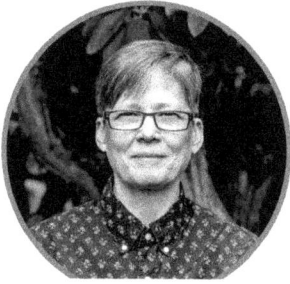

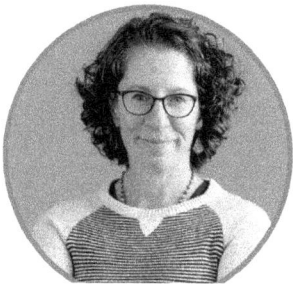

Alex Alexander, ND LMHC

Yes, I once had a person who regularly smoked pot before our sessions. I felt as though we could not connect very well during those sessions. They seemed like a waste of her money and my time. So I asked her to go see someone who might be able to work more directly with her on the situation that was causing her to use drugs to deal with everyday circumstances in life, as this was not my specialty. I also referred two other people to an eating disorder therapist. I felt the work we were doing was secondary to getting deeper work done on the root of their current and past challenges. Again, this is out of my domain of practice. Though I can help if the original symptoms are not acute, and preventing them from focusing on the future in a holistic way.

Tracy Rekart

Ask the Pros

Is there a particular pain-condition or variety of pain that you enjoy working with/have good success with? If so, please elaborate.

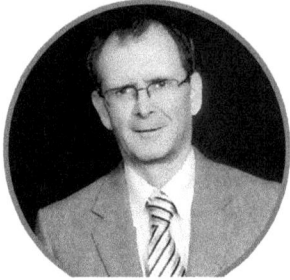

Mark Grant, MA

Fibromyalgia. Because it is a pain disorder with a significant psychological component, as well as physiological stress-related changes. If the client's nervous system can be restored to a less stressed level of functioning, using methods such as EMDR, it is often possible for them to achieve a sense of well-being that is significantly better than before. This often involves treatment of unresolved trauma and its effects (e.g., negative beliefs such as "I am not important"). I often see a dissociation between cognitive and sensory/emotional parts of the personality, which drives a lifestyle that is too goal-focused at the expense of the individual's health and well-being, and I address this with parts work and EMDR aimed at neutralizing the unhealthy emotional drivers and facilitating a more balanced sense of self.

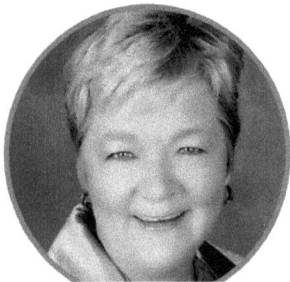

Ilene Dillon, MSW

Emotional pain—not physical (unless emotional pain results in physical pain, which it often does). My focus is on resistance a client might have. Dissolving resistance—whether emotional or physical—can reduce pain. Helping a person to normalize his or her reactions has also been helpful.

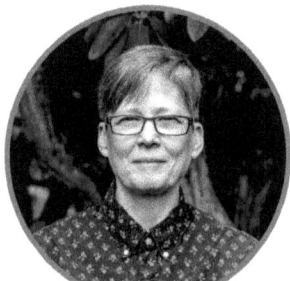

Alex Alexander, ND LMHC

I do well with middle-aged ladies in chronic pain like fibromyalgia who have co-occurring mental health concerns such as anxiety, depression, trauma history, etc. I also do well with cranky men who think anything other than drugs and surgery is dumb. I use a fair bit of manual medicine with those groups, coupled with counseling. It seems to move mountains.

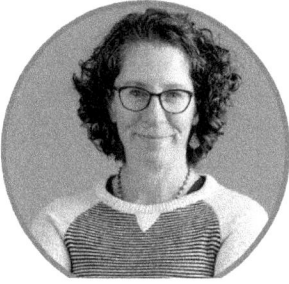

Tracy Rekart

Lower back pain often gets relief in bodywork sessions with me. People generally feel more relaxed and present in their bodies. They often say they can move more freely and easily and feel more settled in themselves. People generally don't come to me with pain, but pain gets resolved through our sessions. An indirect benefit!

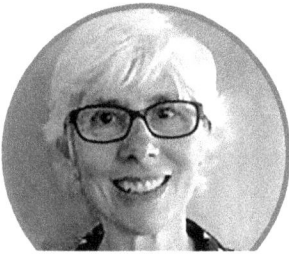

Barbara Rose
Chateaubriand, MA

No.

Ask the Pros

Do you feel that your area of expertise (in regard to pain) relates in some way directly or indirectly to patients' experience of inflammation? If so, how?

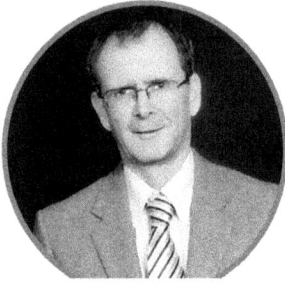

Some recent theories of chronic pain posit that inflammation plays a role, not just the inflammation associated with initial injury, but inflammation associated with stress and aging. If inflammation is partly maintained by stress, then psychological approaches that ameliorate the effects of stress, such as EMDR, meditation, etc., could have an important role to play, as well as providing a rationale for employing non-medical strategies for something which has been traditionally regarded as a medical phenomenon.

Mark Grant, MA

I believe that trauma and the ongoing release of stress hormones correlate with many health conditions that are inflammatory. The inflammation is not my area, but helping with PTSD symptoms, ongoing anxiety, etc., can help to decrease ongoing cortisol release, and hence help with inflammation.

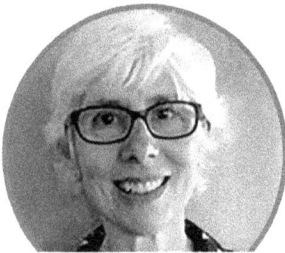

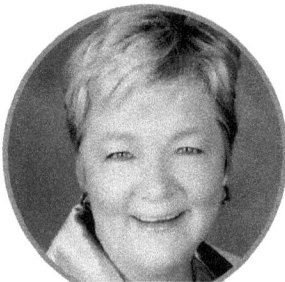

Barbara Rose
Chateaubriand, MA

I think at the root of all human ills is an emotion, especially non-forgiveness.

Ilene Dillon, MSW

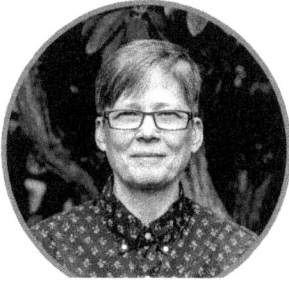

Alex Alexander, ND LMHC

The short answer at face value is "yes." I contribute to inflammation with both manual medicine and counseling services, actually. Let's say I place a gentle force into a joint to release it, and an emotional response results. Does it create inflammation? Does it relieve inflammation? Is it the emotions or the body causing the inflammation? I hope "yes" and "all of the above" because we need inflammation to bring healing, but inflammation unchecked is harmful. We all know inflammation comes from stress, and we are learning even more about how chronic stress changes immune cell genes, leading to more damaging inflammation. The medicine I provide does impact the patient's experience of inflammation, and sometimes it gets a little worse before it gets better. I want to be a controlled burn inflammatory agent. (Does this thing have a smiley face emoji button?)

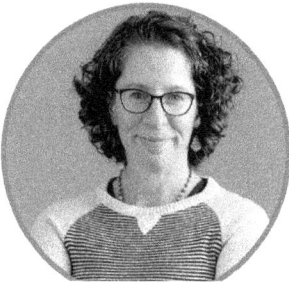

Tracy Rekart

I believe that we armor parts of our body in response to our early learned experiences and how we practiced moving through those with safety, connection, and dignity. This armoring can close us off to parts of ourselves. These closed-off areas have reduced blood flow and attention. When we bring our attention to these places, releases can happen—physically and emotionally. I believe inflammation moves to the areas that we need to tend to. Tending to them may not mean a physical tending, but an emotional or spiritual tending. Something is bringing our attention there; it is a gateway and an invitation to learn about ourselves.

Ask the Pros

Are there common misconceptions about your profession or your work that you encounter with patients? If so, how would you like to see/hear that clarified?

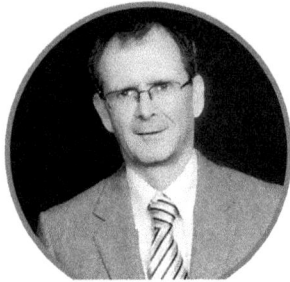

Mark Grant, MA

Mainly, that pain is a physical problem and that non-medical interventions are unlikely to be effective. Along with this, the idea that it is someone else's job (e.g., the doctor) to fix the problem. Also, the idea that if you have to see a psychologist, you must be crazy. There needs to be more recognition that pain is a mind-body problem at all levels of understanding. Amazing how many physicians still dismiss pain for which there is no obvious physical explanation. Given the scientific evidence and the reconceptualization of pain as a mind-body problem, the only explanation for the persistence of the Mind-body split is that it reflects a split in the consciousness of society at large—that we are a dissociated society with an emphasis on doing rather than feeling. McGilchrists 'The Master and His Emissary' looks at the neurological foundations of this in terms of the left and right hemispheres of the brain.

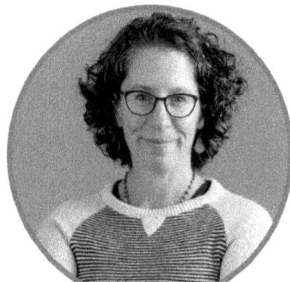

Tracy Rekart

The common misconception when I say I work with and through the body to help people take a balanced stand in their leadership presence is "you work with posture or body language?". Which, in a sense, is true, but really what I work with is the deeper layers of our physiology and psychology and the practices or habits that stem from those patterns. I help shift the body at the level of our early programming, not eradicating that programming, but giving people more choice in the actions they can take. So yes, body language, we can speak more languages. And we also have the competency to listen to more languages, to what people are saying at a deeper level, and connect with people. This leads to sustainable change and more fulfilling, and sometimes challenging relationships. But ultimately, a greater capacity to become who we always knew we could be.

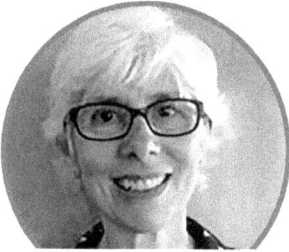

Barbara Rose
Chateaubriand, MA

Many people believe that to acknowledge trauma, especially childhood trauma, it is necessary to blame and judge the people who caused it. Much of the time, the people who created the trauma did so without malintent, and while it is important to make the connections and name cause and effect, it is not necessary to demonize parents and other caregivers.

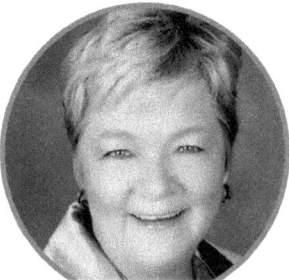

Ilene Dillon, MSW

Not misconceptions about my profession, but often about how I practice within my profession. I want practitioners in my profession to help people look more squarely and realistically at what they are experiencing. I want my fellow professionals to emphasize the need for each person to take personal responsibility for both mental and physical health.

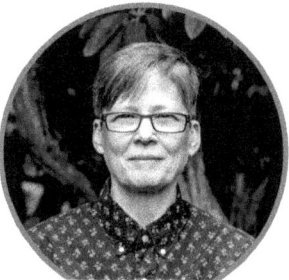

Alex Alexander, ND LMHC

Full disclosure, I don't think most patients know what a naturopathic doctor does since none of us seem to do the same things, so I guess I would say that my flag to carry is that people should know there are licensed and unlicensed naturopathic professionals, and that maybe the licensed ones have more going on educationally and safety-wise. I'm not even sure that is always true, but I'll choose safety in regulation on this one. As for mental health counselors, I think the pack is more homogeneous, and most people know what we do, most probably.

The Take-Aways

➤ An important piece to the experience of any modality is to be shown a way to experience a glimmer of hope …a moment of being pain-free to remind yourself that it's possible.

➤ Find practitioners who will be a sounding board for you and who can help clarify your needs and the path forward for your individual situation.

➤ There seems to be consensus that it takes a village, and not any single modality is the magic bullet. But there also needs to be moderation with the frequency and volume of intervention. One thing at a time and with room in between to let the body rest and process changes.

➤ Sleep, stress management or mitigation, breathing, and eating are things that we all agree will support treatment progress.

➤ Many of us providers take oaths to open our doors to anyone and everyone, but it's natural to develop special interests and strengths for certain types of clinical cases. It's a completely fair question as a patient to inquire about that when interviewing a prospective health-care provider.

➤ Impacting inflammation can happen through many different avenues, but there seems to be some consensus that doing so is directly and indirectly part of care when pain is at play.

➤ As a patient, it might be useful to set aside preconceived notions about certain disciplines of healthcare because no two practitioners deliver the same experience of human interaction. The therapeutic relationship can be as unique as each human being.

Hopefully, these interviews offer you a snapshot of the vast array of biomechanical modalities and their potential benefits to you during times of need. But also, that the reach is wider than just body mechanics.

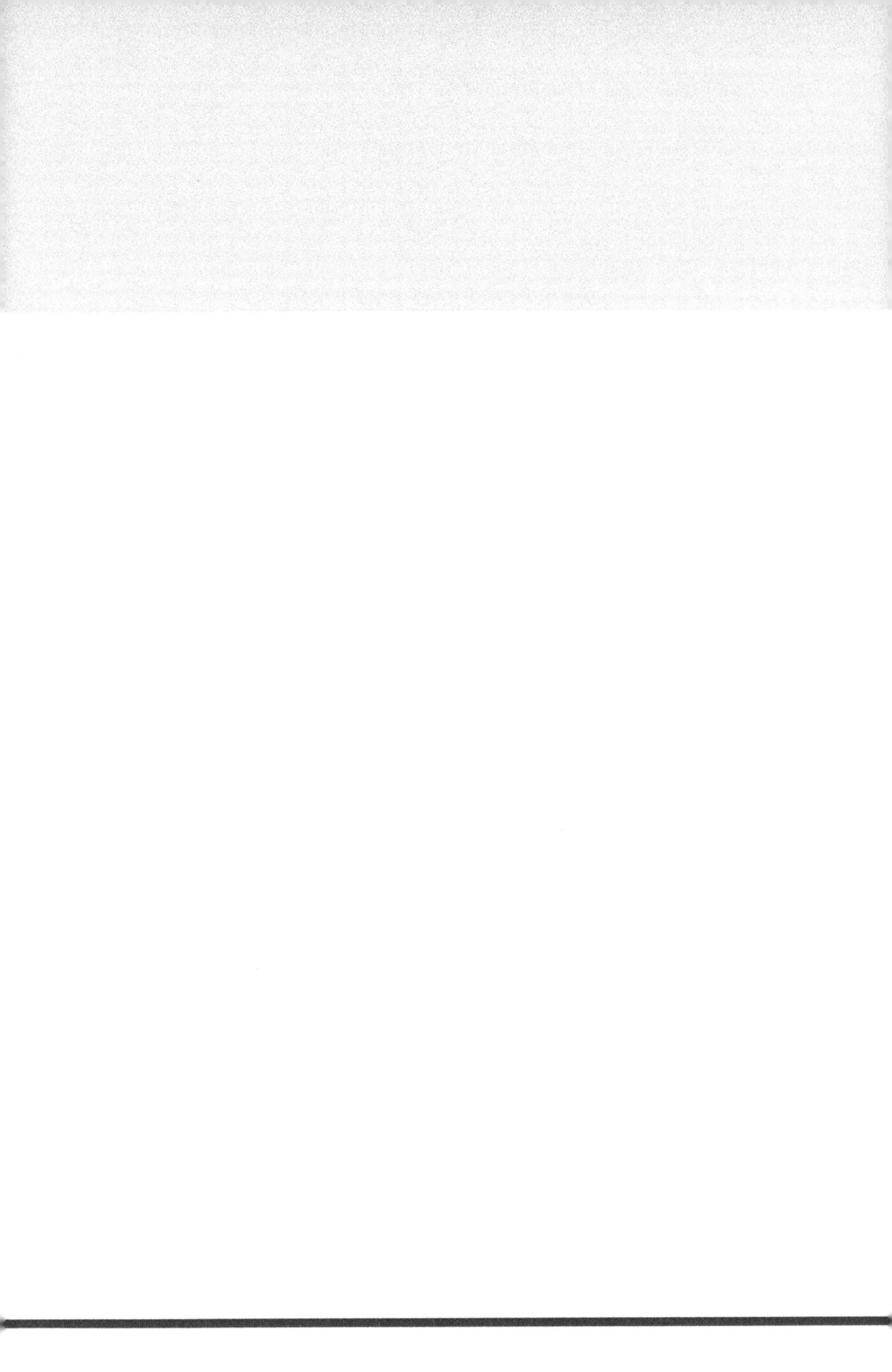

MAKE THE MOST OF YOUR VISIT

Questions to ask when checking out new practitioners to aid with biomechanical reinforcement:

1. How do you see your role in this process?

2. What are your expectations of me?

3. Is there a timeline with milestones to reach for?

4. How do you measure progress, and when do I know it's time to move on?

5. How often do you see and work with clinical cases like mine?

ABOUT THE AUTHOR

YA-LING J. LIOU, DC, is a chiropractic physician who, after more than 30 years of clinical experience, continues to expand and share her intuitive body care techniques. All of her work takes into account the whole person, aiming not only to address the mechanical balance of the body, but also the chemical and emotional aspects that so often influence this balance.

Growing up with exposure to generations of Eastern as well as Western attitudes toward health has provided Dr. Liou with a unique perspective on health care. She began her formal education in the area of applied sciences in her hometown of Montreal, Quebec, before completing a degree program at New York Chiropractic College.

Dr. Liou now lives, works, and writes in Seattle. She taught anatomy, physiology and kinesiology at Seattle Massage School (currently Everest College and formerly Ashmead College) and later brought her multiple-systems perspective to the Naturopathic Physical Medicine Department at Bastyr University as an adjunct faculty member.

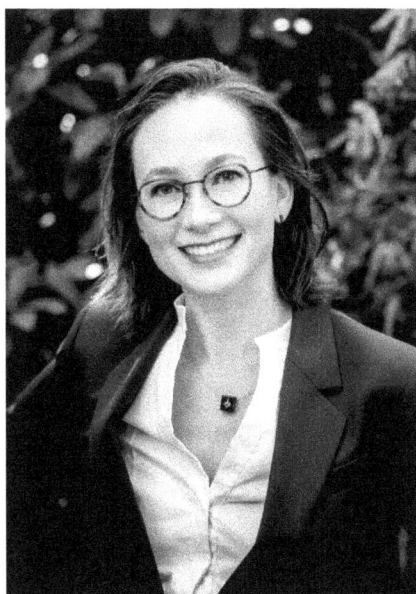

Want to learn more? Stay connected with
the author by visitng www.ya-ling.com.

www.ingramcontent.com/pod-product-compliance
Lightning Source LLC
Chambersburg PA
CBHW051323020426
42333CB00032B/3460